AA

Guide for the Disabled Traveller 1993/94

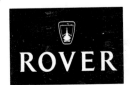

ROVER

Produced by the Publishing Division of the Automobile Association

Consultant Editor: Roy Thompson, MBE

Head of Advertisement Sales: Christopher Heard
Tel (0256) 20123

Advertisement Production: Karen Weeks
Tel (0256) 20123

Directory: Compiled by the AA's Research Unit, Information Control and generated by the AA's Establishment database.

Cover design: Paul Hampson Partnership

Cover photograph: Gordon Hammond ABIPP, Southampton

Graphic design: Peter C. Gibbons

Typeset by: Microset Graphics Ltd, Basingstoke

Printed by: BPCC Wheatons Ltd, Exeter

Published by the Automobile Association
Fanum House, Basingstoke, Hampshire RG21 2EA

ISBN 0-7495-0637-7

CONTENTS

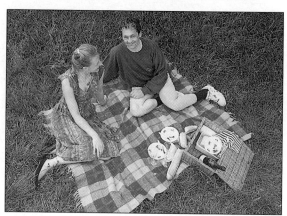

GUIDE FOR THE DISABLED TRAVELLER

INTRODUCTION BY THE EARL OF SNOWDON GCVO

There are 6 million people with a mobility handicap in the United Kingdom. They form 10 per cent of the population. Yet all too often they continue to be a forgotten minority.

Why?

It takes little more than forethought to ensure that facilities are in place to enable people with disabilities to participate more fully in everyday life.

Town planners, architects, transport managers . . . there is a responsibility on anyone who designs or manages amenities that are open to the public to ensure that they are accessible to **everyone.**

Progress **is** *being made. Increasingly, it is realised that facilities that make life easier for people with a mobility handicap make life easier for everyone else too. But there is still a long way to go before a substantial number of people in our country can travel in comfort and with confidence.*

I welcome publication of this latest edition of the Guide for the Disabled Traveller. Since the AA first published the Guide in the late 1960s, its information has helped considerably to break down the barrier of apprehension about what may await the disabled traveller at the end of his or her journey.

As a result, it continues to be an invaluable aid to those who seek no more than a right that most of us take for granted: the right to travel.

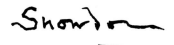

FOREWORD

WITHOUT confidence many people with disabilities would never travel.

I recently visited a town that has been pedestrianised. Although this should have made it easier to get around in my wheelchair, there were no parking spaces near to the shops for disabled people so I couldn't get anywhere near a shop that I have visited for years. A special disabled person's parking permit had also been introduced – absolutely useless for visitors to the town who didn't have it!

The contrast to a second shopping area that has joined the "Shopmobility scheme" could not have been greater. There was a free, Shopmobility car park, and a safe "drop-off" point for anyone arriving in the town by car or taxi. There were helpers on hand and wheelchairs or scooters that could be hired. The whole area was designed with disabled people in mind.

These two examples show very clearly the difference that confidence can make. On the first trip, I had to abandon my journey without achieving what I needed – simply because I wasn't confident that I could get to the shops. In the second example, I knew that I would be able to park near to the stores and use ramps instead of steps – much easier, incidentally, for mothers with prams as well as for people in wheelchairs.

This latest edition of the *Guide for the Disabled Traveller* is all about giving people the information and the confidence they need to travel – including a list of towns with a Shopmobility scheme.

Roy Thompson MBE
The AA's Disability Consultant

PLACES TO VISIT

The following places to visit have been selected from the AA's publication *2000 Days Out in Britain*. The properties have not been inspected but proprietors have indicated that their establishments are accessible to visitors in wheelchairs. It is advisable to check with the establishment concerned before making a visit.

Full details of each property, including admission prices, and opening dates, are included in *2000 Days Out in Britain,* available from AA shops and major booksellers.

ACCESS FOR ALL WITH THE NATIONAL TRUST

The National Trust is a charity which protects about 650,000 acres of beautiful coast and countryside in England, Wales and Northern Ireland, open to countless millions of visitors each year. It opens some 300 houses, castles and gardens to the public, and welcomes to these more than 10 million people annually. The Trust has well over two million members.

With all these visitors it's not surprising that great care is taken to welcome and provide comfortable and enjoyable visits for people with disabilities of all kinds. The Trust estimates that between 20 and 25 per cent of its members and visitors have a disability or infirmity. It tries wherever possible to provide opportunities for all its visitors to integrate and enjoy Trust properties together – to this end, self-drive and volunteer-driven buggies and other powered vehicles are increasingly used in National Trust gardens and parks.

The Trust has ten adapted holiday cottages in England and Northern Ireland; it is introducing the Sympathetic Hearing Scheme at a growing number of properties and recommends gardens and countryside with scented plants, sounds and textures for visually impaired visitors to enjoy. Braille guides are supplied free.

Drivers may set down disabled passengers near the entrance to a house or garden, and disabled drivers may park as close to a property as space permits, but they are encouraged to telephone ahead of a visit to ensure this provision is available.

The necessary companion of a disabled visitor is given free admission on request.

Properties administered by the National Trust have been highlighted in the following list (NT). For further information regarding any of these properties please contact: Valerie Wenham, The National Trust, 36 Queen Anne's Gate, London SW1H 9AS *tel* 071-222 9251.

ENGLAND

AVON

Bath
Holburne Museum & Crafts Study Centre
tel (0225) 466669
The Royal Photographic Society
tel (0225) 462841

Bristol
Bristol Industrial Museum *tel* (0272) 251470
Maritime Heritage Centre *tel* (0272) 260680

The Exploratory Hands-on-Science Centre
tel (0272) 252008

Dyrham
Dyrham Park *tel* (027582) 2501 ♨ *(NT)*

Weston-super-Mare
International Helicopter Museum
tel (0934) 635227

BEDFORDSHIRE

Bedford
Bedford Museum *tel* (0234) 353323

Cecil Higgins Art Gallery & Museum
tel (0234) 211222

Old Warden
The Shuttleworth Collection *tel* (076727) 288

Whipsnade
Whipsnade Wild Animal Park
tel (0582) 872171

Woburn
Woburn Wild Animal Kingdom & Leisure Park
tel (0525) 290407 ᎬᎬ

BERKSHIRE

Basildon
Basildon Park *tel* (0734) 843040 ᎬᎬ *(NT)*
Beale Bird Park
tel (0491) 671325 or (0734) 845172 ᎬᎬ

Maidenhead
Courage Shire Horse Centre
tel (062882) 4848 ᎬᎬ

Reading
Blake's Lock Museum *tel* (0734) 390918

Riseley
Wellington Country Park & National Dairy
Museum *tel* (0734) 326444

Windsor
Exhibition of the Queen's Presents & Royal
Carriages *tel* (0753) 831118
Household Cavalry Museum
tel (0735) 868222 *ext* 5203
Royalty & Empire Exhibition
tel (0753) 857837
Savill Garden (Windsor Great Park)
tel (0753) 860222
St. George's Chapel *tel* (0753) 865538 ᎬᎬ
State Apartments *tel* (0753) 831118
Valley Gardens (Windsor Great Park)
tel (0753) 860222

BUCKINGHAMSHIRE

Aylesbury
Buckinghamshire County Museum
tel (0296) 88849

Beaconsfield
Bekonscot Model Village
tel (0494) 672919

Chalfont St Giles
Milton's Cottage *tel* (02407) 213 ᎬᎬ

Cliveden
Cliveden *tel* (0628) 605069 ᎬᎬ *(NT)*

Hughenden
Hughenden Manor *tel* (0494) 532580 ᎬᎬ *(NT)*

Middle Claydon
Claydon House *tel* (0296) 730349 ᎬᎬ *(NT)*

Quainton
Buckinghamshire Railway Centre
tel (029675) 720 ᎬᎬ

Stowe
Stowe Landscaped Gardens
tel (0280) 822850 ᎬᎬ *(NT)*

Waddesdon
Waddesdon Manor *tel* (0296) 651211 ᎬᎬ *(NT)*

CAMBRIDGESHIRE

Cambridge
Fitzwilliam Museum *tel* (0223) 332900
University Botanic Garden *tel* (0223) 336265
University Museum of Archaeology &
Anthropology *tel* (0223) 337733

Linton
Linton Zoological Gardens *tel* (0223) 891308

Lode
Anglesey Abbey *tel* (0223) 811200 ᎬᎬ *(NT)*

Peakirk
Wildfowl & Wetlands Trust *tel* (0733) 252271

St Ives
Norris Museum *tel* (0480) 65101

Wansford
Nene Valley Railway *tel* (0780) 782854 ᎬᎬ

Wimpole
Wimpole Hall *tel* (0223) 207257 ᎬᎬ *(NT)*
Wimpole Home Farm *tel* (0223) 207257 ᎬᎬ *(NT)*

CHESHIRE

Chester
Chester Zoo *tel* (0244) 380280

Disley
Lyme Park *tel* (0663) 762023 ❄ *(NT)*

Ellesmere Port
Boat Museum *tel* 051-355 5017

Jodrell Bank
Jodrell Bank Science Centre & Arboretum
tel (0477) 71339

Knutsford
Tatton Park *tel* (0565) 654822 ❄ *(NT)*

Macclesfield
Macclesfield Silk Museum *tel* (0625) 613210
West Park Museum *tel* (0625) 619831

Nantwich
Stapeley Water Gardens
tel (0270) 623868 & 628628

Scholar Green
Little Moreton Hall *tel* (0260) 272018 ❄ *(NT)*

Styal
Quarry Bank Mill & Styal Country Park
tel (0625) 527468 *(NT)*

Widnes
Catalyst – The Museum of the Chemical Industry
tel 051-420 1121

CLEVELAND

Guisborough
Gisborough Priory *tel* (0287) 38301

Middlesbrough
Captain Cook Birthplace Museum
tel (0642) 311211

Ormesby
Ormesby Hall *tel* (0642) 324188 ❄ *(NT)*

CO DURHAM

Barnard Castle
Bowes Museum *tel* (0833) 690606
Egglestone Abbey

Darlington
Darlington Railway Centre & Museum
tel (0325) 460532

❄ *Seasonal Opening*
(NT) National Trust

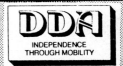

Durham
Durham Light Infantry Museum & Arts Centre
tel 091-384 2214
Finchale Priory *tel* 091-386 3828

CORNWALL & ISLES OF SCILLY

Calstock
Cotehele *tel* (0579) 50434 & 51222 ୬ᵉ *(NT)*

Dobwalls
Thorburn Museum & Gallery
tel (0579) 20325 & 21129

Goonhavern
World in Miniature *tel* (0872) 572828 ୬ᵉ

Gweek
Seal Sanctuary & Marine Animal Rescue Centre
tel (032622) 361

Helston
Flambards Village Theme Park *tel* (0326) 573404
& 574549 ୬ᵉ
Helston Folk Museum
tel (03265) 564027 & 561672

Lanhydrock *tel* (0208) 73320 *(NT)*

Lanreath
Lanreath Farm & Folk Museum
tel (0503) 20321 ୬ᵉ

Looe
Monkey Sanctuary *tel* (05036) 2532 ୬ᵉ

Madron
Trengwainton Garden *tel* (0736) 63021 ୬ᵉ *(NT)*

Mevagissey
World of Model Railways
tel (0726) 842457 ୬ᵉ

Newquay
Dairyland *tel* (0872) 510246 ୬ᵉ

St Austell
Charlestown Shipwreck & Heritage Museum
tel (0726) 69897 ୬ᵉ

Tredinnick
Cornish Shire Horse Centre
tel (0841) 540276 ୬ᵉ

Trelissick Garden
tel (0872) 862090 & 865808 ୬ᵉ *(NT)*

Trerice *tel* (0637) 875404 ୬ᵉ *(NT)*

Truro
Royal Cornwall Museum *tel* (0872) 72205

CUMBRIA

Barrow-in-Furness
Furness Abbey *tel* (0229) 823420

Brampton
Lanercrost Priory *tel* (06977) 3030 ୬ᵉ

Grizedale
Visitor Centre *tel* (0229) 860373 ୬ᵉ

Kendal
Kendal Museum *tel* (0539) 721374

Keswick
Cars of the Stars Motor Museum
tel (07687) 73757 ୬ᵉ

Millom
Millom Folk Museum *tel* (0229) 772555 ୬ᵉ

Ravenglass
Ravenglass & Eskdale Railway
tel (0229) 717171 ୬ᵉ

Sedbergh
National Park Centre *tel* (05396) 20125

Shap
Shap Abbey

Sizergh
Sizergh Castle Garden *tel* (05395) 60070 ୬ᵉ *(NT)*

Temple Sowerby
Acorn Bank Garden *tel* (07683) 61893 ୬ᵉ *(NT)*

Ulverston
Laurel & Hardy Museum
tel (0229) 52292 & 861614

Windermere
Windermere Steamboat Museum
tel (05394) 45565 ୬ᵉ

DERBYSHIRE

Bolsover
Bolsover Castle *tel* (0246) 823349

Buxton
Buxton Micrarium *tel* (0298) 78662 ୬ᵉ

Calke
Calke Abbey *tel* (0332) 863822 ୬ᵉ *(NT)*

Creswell
Creswell Crags Visitor Centre
tel (0909) 720378

Crich
National Tramway Museum
tel (0773) 852565 ☀

Derby
Derby Pottery Visitors Centre *tel* (0773) 743644
Derby Museum & Art Gallery *tel* (0332) 255586 & 255587
Industrial Museum *tel* (0332) 293111 *ext* 740

Hardwick Hall *tel* (0246) 850340 ☀ *(NT)*

Ilkeston
The American Adventure
tel (0773) 769931 & 531521 ☀

Kedleston Hall *tel* (0332) 842191 ☀ *(NT)*

Lea
Lea Gardens *tel* (0629) 534380 ☀

Matlock
Riber Castle Wildlife Park *tel* (0629) 582073

Sudbury
Sudbury Hall *tel* (0283) 585305 ☀ *(NT)*

DEVON

Arlington
Arlington Court *tel* (0271) 850296 ☀ *(NT)*

Beer
Pecorama Pleasure Gardens *tel* (0297) 21542

Bickington
Gorse Blossom Miniature Railway and Woodland Park *tel* (0626) 821361 ☀

Bicton
Bicton Park Gardens *tel* (0395) 68465 ☀

Blackmoor Gate
Exmoor Bird Gardens *tel* (05983) 352

Buckfastleigh
Buckfast Abbey *tel* (0364) 42519
Buckfast Butterfly Farm & Dartmoor Otter Sanctuary *tel* (0364) 42916 ☀
South Devon Railway *tel* (0364) 42338 ☀

Buckland Abbey *tel* (0822) 853607 *(NT)*

Combe Martin
The Combe Martin Motorcycle Collection
tel (0271) 882346 ☀

Dartmouth
Woodland Leisure Park *tel* (080421) 598

Drewsteignton
Castle Drogo *tel* (0647) 433306 ☀ *(NT)*

Great Torrington
RHS Garden Rosemoor *tel* (0805) 24067

Ilfracombe
Ilfracombe Museum *tel* (0271) 863541

Killerton House & Garden *tel* (0392) 881345 *(NT)*

Knightshayes Court *tel* (0884) 254665 ☀ *(NT)*

Paignton
Paignton & Dartmouth Steam Railway
tel (0803) 555872 ☀
Zoological & Botanical Gardens
tel (0803) 527936

Plymouth
City Museum & Art Gallery
tel (0752) 264878
Plymouth Dome *tel* (0752) 603300 & 600608

Plympton
Dartmoor Wildlife Park & Westcountry Falconry Centre *tel* (075537) 209 & 343

Torquay
Babbacombe Model Village *tel* (0803) 328669
Kents Cavern Showcaves *tel* (0803) 294059 & 215136

Yealmpton
The National Shire Horse Centre
tel (0752) 880268

Yelverton
Paperweight Centre *tel* (0822) 854250

DORSET

Abbotsbury
Abbotsbury Sub Tropical Gardens
tel (0305) 871387
Abbotsbury Swannery
tel (0305) 871242 & 871684

Bournemouth
The Shelley Rooms *tel* (0202) 303571

Canford Cliffs
Compton Acres Gardens *tel* (0202) 700778 ☀

Corfe Castle
Corfe Castle Museum *tel* (0929) 480415

☀ *Seasonal Opening*
(NT) National Trust

Dorchester
Tutankhamun Exhibition *tel* (0305) 269571

Poole
Waterfront Museum *tel* (0202) 683138

Shaftesbury
Abbey Ruins & Museum *tel* (0747) 52910 ✵

Sherborne
Sherborne Old Castle *tel* (0935) 812730

Swanage
Swanage Railway *tel* (0929) 425800 & 424276
(timetable)

Verwood
Dorset Heavy Horse Centre
tel (0202) 824040 ✵

Weymouth
Sea Life Park *tel* (0305) 788255
The Deep Sea Adventure & Titanic Story
tel (0305) 760690

Wimborne
Knoll Gardens *tel* (0202) 873931 ✵

EAST SUSSEX

Alfriston
Drusillas Park *tel* (0323) 870234

Bexhill
Bexhill Museum of Costume & Social History
tel (0424) 215361 ✵

Bodiam
Bodiam Castle *tel* (058083) 436 *(NT)*

Brighton
Sea Life Centre *tel* (0273) 604233 & 604234

Eastbourne
Eastbourne Redoubt Fortress
tel (0323) 410300 ✵

Exceat
The Living World *tel* (0323) 870100

Halland
Bentley Wildfowl & Motor Museum
tel (0825) 840573

Hastings
Hastings Embroidery *tel* (0424) 718888

Pevensey
Pevensey Castle *tel* (0323) 762604

Sheffield Park
Sheffield Park Garden
tel (0825) 790655 ✵ *(NT)*

ESSEX

Coggleshall
Paycocke's *tel* (0376) 561305 ✵ *(NT)*

Colchester
Colchester Zoo *tel* (0839) 222000
Natural History Museum *tel* (0206) 712931
Trinity Museum *tel* (0206) 712931
Tymperleys Clock Museum
tel (0206) 712931 & 712932 ✵

Grays
Thurrock Museum *tel* (0375) 390000 *ext.* 2414

Harlow
Mark Hall Cycle Museum & Gardens
tel (0279) 39680

Waltham Abbey
Hayes Hill Farm *tel* (099289) 2291

GLOUCESTERSHIRE

Bourton-on-the-Water
Birdland *tel* (0451) 20689 & 20480
Cotswold Motor Museum *tel* (0451) 21255 ✵
Folly Farm Waterfowl *tel* (0451) 20285

Chedworth
Roman Villa *tel* (024289) 256 ✵ *(NT)*

Cheltenham
Art Gallery & Museum *tel* (0242) 237431

Cirencester
Corinium Museum *tel* (0285) 655611

Cranham
Prinknash Abbey *tel* (0452) 812239

Gloucester
City Museum & Art Gallery *tel* (0452) 524131
National Waterways Museum
tel (0452) 307009
The Robert Opie Collection-Museum of
Packaging & Advertising *tel* (0452) 302309

Great Witcombe
Witcombe Roman Villa

Guiting Power
Cotswold Farm Park *tel* (0451) 850307 ✵

Hailes
Hailes Abbey *tel* (0242) 602398

Lydney
Dean Forest Railway *tel* (0594) 843423

Mickleton
Hidcote Manor Garden *tel* (0386) 438333 🌂 *(NT)*

Moreton-in-Marsh
Cotswold Falconry Centre *tel* (0386) 701043 🌂

Newent
The National Birds of Prey Centre
tel (0531) 820286 🌂

Northleach
Keith Harding's World of Mechanical Music
tel (0451) 60181

Slimbridge
Wildfowl & Wetlands Trust *tel* (0453) 890333

Twigworth
Nature in Art *tel* (0452) 731422

Westbury-on-Severn
Westbury Court Garden *tel* (045276) 461 🌂 *(NT)*

Westonbirt
Westonbirt Arboretum *tel* (066688) 220

GREATER MANCHESTER

Altrincham
Dunham Massey Hall *tel* 061-941 1025 🌂 *(NT)*

Ashton-Under-Lyne
Museum of the Manchesters *tel* 061-344 3078
Portland Basin Industrial Heritage Centre
tel 061-308 3374

Bolton
Tonge Moor Textile Museum *tel* (0204) 21394

Manchester
Granada Studio Tours
tel 061-833 0880 & 061-832 9090
Manchester Museum *tel* 061-275 2634
Manchester Museum of Transport
tel 061-205 2122 & 061-205 1082
Manchester United Museum & Tour Centre
tel 061-877 4002
Whitworth Art Gallery
tel 061-273 5958 & 061-273 4865

Salford
Salford Museum & Art Gallery *tel* 061-736 2649

HAMPSHIRE

Aldershot
Airborne Forces Museum *tel* (0252) 349619

Alresford
Mid Hants Railway
tel (0962) 733810 & 734200 🌂

Ampfield
Hillier Gardens & Arboretum *tel* (0794) 68787

Andover
Finkley Down Farm Park *tel* (0264) 352195 🌂

Ashurst
New Forest Butterfly Farm *tel* (0703) 292166 🌂

Burghclere
Sandham Memorial Chapel
tel (063527) 292 *(NT)*

East Tisted
Rotherfield Park *tel* (042058) 204 🌂

Hinton Ampner *tel* (0372) 53401 🌂 *(NT)*

Liphook
Bohunt Manor *tel* (0428) 722208

Lyndhurst
New Forest Museum & Visitor Centre
tel (0703) 283914

Marwell
Marwell Zoological Park
tel Owslebury (0962) 777406

Middle Wallop
Museum of Army Flying *tel* (0264) 384421

Mottisfont
Mottisfont Abbey Garden *tel* (0794) 41220 &
40757 🌂 *(NT)*

Netley
Netley Abbey *tel* (0703) 453076

New Milton
Sammy Miller Museum *tel* (0425) 619696

Ower
Paultons Park *tel* (0703) 814455 🌂

Portsmouth
D-Day Museum & Overlord Embroidery
tel (0705) 827261
The Mary Rose Ship Hall & Exhibition
tel (0705) 839766 & 750521

🌂 *Seasonal Opening*
(NT) National Trust

13

Rockbourne
Roman Villa *tel* (07253) 541 ৠ

Sherborne St John
The Vyne *tel* (0256) 881337 ৠ *(NT)*

Southampton
Southampton City Art Gallery
tel (0703) 231375
Southampton Hall of Aviation
tel (0703) 635830

Stratfield Saye
Stratfield Saye House *tel* (0256) 882882 ৠ

Weyhill
The Hawk Conservancy *tel* (0264) 772252 ৠ

Winchester
Guildhall Gallery *tel* (0962) 848296 & 52874
Gurkha Museum *tel* (0962) 842832
Royal Hussars Regimental Museum
tel (0962) 863751
The Great Hall of Winchester Castle
tel (0962) 846476

HEREFORD & WORCESTER

Ashton
Berrington Hall *tel* (0568) 615721 ৠ *(NT)*

Bewdley
Bewdley Museum *tel* (0299) 403573 ৠ
West Midland Safari & Leisure Park
tel (0299) 402114 ৠ

Brockhampton
Lower Brockhampton ৠ

Croft
Croft Castle *tel* (056885) 246 ৠ *(NT)*

Hanbury
Hanbury Hall *tel* (052784) 214 ৠ *(NT)*

Hereford
Hereford Museum & Art Gallery
tel (0432) 268121 *ext* 207

Ross-On-Wye
The Lost Street Museum *tel* ((0989) 62752

Spetchley
Spetchley Park Gardens
tel (090565) 213 or 224 ৠ

Stone
Stone House Cottage Gardens
tel (0562) 69902 ৠ

Symonds Yat (West)
The Jubilee Park *tel* (0600) 890360

Worcester
City Museum & Art Gallery *tel* (0905) 25371
Dyson Perrins Museum *tel* (0905) 23221

HERTFORDSHIRE

Berkhamsted
Berkhamsted Castle

Hatfield
Hatfield House *tel* (0707) 262823 ৠ

St Albans
Roman Theatre of Verulamium *tel* (0727) 835035
St Albans Organ Museum *tel* (0727) 869693
The Gardens of the Rose (Royal National Rose
Society) *tel* (0727) 50461 ৠ
Verulamium Museum *tel* (0727) 819339 ৠ

Stevenage
Stevenage Museum *tel* (0438) 354292

Watford
Watford Museum *tel* (0923) 32297

HUMBERSIDE

Grimsby
National Fishing Heritage Centre
tel (0472) 242000
Welholme Galleries *tel* (0472) 242000 *ext* 1385

Hornsea
Hornsea Pottery & Leisure Park
tel (0964) 534211

Hull
Town Docks Museum *tel* (0482) 593902

KENT

Aylesford
Aylesford Priory *tel* (0622) 717272

Bekesbourne
Howletts Zoo Park *tel* (0227) 721286

Borough Green
Great Comp Garden *tel* (0732) 882669 ৠ

Brasted
Emmett's Garden *tel* (073275) 367 ৠ *(NT)*

Canterbury
Blean Bird Park *tel* (0227) 471666 ৠ
The Canterbury Tales *tel* (0227) 454888

Chartwell *tel* (0732) 866368 ❄ *(NT)*

Dover
The White Cliffs Experience *tel* (0304) 214566

Eynsford
Eynsford Castle *tel* (0322) 862536

Gillingham
Royal Engineers Museum *tel* (0634) 406397

Hawkinge
Kent Battle of Britain Museum
tel (030389) 3140 ❄

Herne Common
'Brambles' Wildlife Park *tel* (0227) 712379 ❄

Ightham
Ightham Mote *tel* (0732) 810378 ❄ *(NT)*

Lamberhurst
Bayham Priory *tel* (0892) 890381 ❄

Richborough
Richborough Castle *tel* (0304) 612013

Royal Tunbridge Wells
Tunbridge Wells Museum & Art Gallery
tel (0892) 526121 *ext* 3171

Sissinghurst
Sissinghurst Castle Garden
tel (0580) 712850 ❄ *(NT)*

LANCASHIRE

Blackpool
Zoological Gardens *tel* (0253) 65027

Charnock Richard
Camelot Theme Park *tel* (0257) 453044 ❄

Lancaster
Maritime Museum *tel* (0524) 64637

Leyland
British Commercial Vehicle Museum
tel (0772) 451011 ❄

Martin Mere
Wildfowl & Wetlands Trust *tel* (0704) 895181

Rufford
Rufford Old Hall *tel* (0704) 821254 ❄ *(NT)*

Whalley
Whalley Abbey *tel* (0254) 822268

❄ *Seasonal Opening*
(NT) National Trust

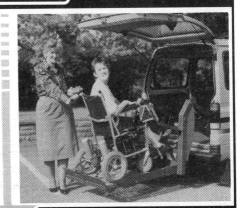
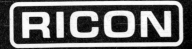

LEICESTERSHIRE

Cottesmore
Rutland Railway Museum
tel (0780) 62384 & 63092 ☼

Leicester
Leicestershire Museum & Art Gallery
tel (0533) 554100
Leicestershire Record Office
tel (0533) 544566

Market Bosworth
Bosworth Battlefield Visitor Centre &
Country Park *tel* (0455) 290429
The Battlefield Steam Railway Line
tel (0827) 880754 & (0827) 715790 (weekends)

Market Harborough
Harborough Museum *tel* (0858) 32468

Oakham
Oakham Castle *tel* (0572) 723654

LINCOLNSHIRE

Belton
Belton House Park & Garden
tel (0476) 66116 ☼ *(NT)*

Coningsby
Battle of Britain Memorial Flight Visitor Centre
tel (0526) 44041

Lincoln
National Cycle Museum *tel* (0522) 545091
Usher Gallery *tel* (0522) 27980

Skegness
Skegness Natureland Marine Zoo
tel (0754) 764345

Spalding
Butterfly & Falconry Park *tel* (0406) 363833 ☼
Springfield Gardens *tel* (0775) 724843 ☼

Tattershall
Tattershall Castle *tel* (0526) 42543 ☼ *(NT)*

LONDON (Central)

E2
Bethnal Green Museum of Childhood
tel 081-980 2415 & 081-980 3204

E6
East Ham Nature Reserve *tel* 081-470 4525

EC2
Museum of London
tel 071-600 3699 *ext* 240 or 280

NW1
Madame Tussaud's *tel* 071-935 6861

NW9
Royal Air Force Museum *tel* 081-205 2266

SE1
Florence Nightingale Museum *tel* 071-620 0374
Imperial War Museum *tel* 071-416 5000
Museum of the Moving Image *tel* 071-401 2636
Museum of Garden History
tel 071-261 1891 (between 11am-3pm) ☼
The Design Museum at Butler's Wharf
tel 071-403 6933
The London Dungeon *tel* 071-403 0606
Tower Bridge *tel* 071-407 0922 & 071-407 5247

SE21
Dulwich Picture Gallery *tel* 081-693 5254

SW1
Cabinet War Rooms *tel* 071-930 6961
Royal Mews *tel* 071-799 2331
Tate Gallery *tel* 071-821 1313 & 071-821 7128

SW3
National Army Museum *tel* 071-730 0717

SW7
Natural History Museum *tel* 071-938 9123
Science Museum *tel* 071-938 8000

SW19
Wimbledon Lawn Tennis Museum
tel 081-946 6131

W1
Guinness World of Records Exhibitions
tel 071-439 7331
Museum of Mankind *tel* 071-636 1555 *ext* 8043
Rock Circus *tel* 071-734 7203
Royal Academy of Arts *tel* 071-439 7438
Wallace Collection *tel* 071-935 0687

W8
Commonwealth Institute *tel* 071-603 4535

WC1
The Jewish Museum *tel* 071-388 4525

WC2
Courtauld Institute Galleries *tel* 071-873 2526
London Transport Museum *tel* 071-379 6344

National Gallery *tel* 071-839 3321
Theatre Museum *tel* 071-836 7891

LONDON (Greater)

Chislehurst
Chislehurst Caves *tel* 081-467 3264

Ham
Ham House *tel* 081-940 1950 ✹ *(NT)*

Isleworth
Heritage Motor Museum (Syon Park)
tel 081-560 1378
Syon House *tel* 081-560 0881/3 ✹

Osterley
Osterley Park House *tel* 081-560 3918 ✹ *(NT)*

MERSEYSIDE

Birkenhead
Williamson Art Gallery & Museum
tel 051-652 4177

Liverpool
Animation World *tel* 051-707 1828
Liverpool Football Club Visitors Centre
tel 051-263 2361
Liverpool Libraries & Arts *tel* 051-225 5429
Merseyside Maritime Museum *tel* 051-207 0001
Museum of Labour History
tel 051-207 0001 *ext* 279
Tate Gallery *tel* 051-709 0507
The Beatles Story *tel* 051-709 1963

Port Sunlight
Port Sunlight Heritage Centre *tel* 051-644 6466

Prescot
Knowsley Safari Park *tel* 051-430 9009 ✹

Southport
Atkinson Art Gallery *tel* (0704) 533133 *ext* 2111
Southport Railway Centre *tel* (0704) 530693
Southport Zoo *tel* (0704) 538102

Speke
Speke Hall *tel* 051-427 7231 ✹ *(NT)*

St Helens
Pilkington Glass Museum
tel (0744) 692499 & 692014

NORFOLK

Banham
Banham Zoo & Appleyard Craft Court
tel (095387) 771

Blickling
Blickling Hall *tel* (0263) 733084 ✹ *(NT)*

Cromer
Lifeboat Museum *tel* (0263) 512503 ✹

Felbrigg
Felbrigg Hall *tel* (026375) 444 ✹ *(NT)*

Filby
Thrigby Hall Wildlife Gardens *tel* (0493) 369477

Glandford
Shell Museum *tel* (0263) 740081

Great Yarmouth
Merrivale Model Village *tel* (0493) 842097 ✹
Museum Exhibition Galleries *tel* (0493) 858900

Gressenhall
Gressenhall Rural Life Museum & Union Farm
tel (0362) 860563 ✹

Heacham
Norfolk Lavender *tel* (0485) 70384

Houghton
Houghton Hall *tel* (048522) 569 ✹

King's Lynn
Lynn Museum *tel* (0553) 775001

Little Walsingham
Walsingham Abbey Grounds *tel* (0328) 820259

Norwich
Sainsbury Centre For Visual Arts
tel (0603) 56060 & 592467
St Peter Hungate Church Museum
tel (0603) 667231

Oxborough
Oxburgh Hall *tel* (036621) 258 ✹ *(NT)*

Reedham
Pettitts Feathercraft & Animal Adventure Park
tel (0493) 700094 ✹

Sandringham
Sandringham House, Grounds, Museum &
Country Park *tel* (0553) 772675 ✹
Wolferton Station *tel* (0485) 540674 ✹

Sheringham
North Norfolk Railway *tel* (0263) 822045 ✹

✹ *Seasonal Opening*
(NT) National Trust

South Walsham
The Fairhaven Garden Trust *tel* (060549) 449 ♨

Thetford
Thetford Priory ♨

Thursford Green
Thursford Collection *tel* (0328) 878477 ♨

West Runton
Norfolk Shire Horse Centre *tel* (026375) 339 ♨

NORTH YORKSHIRE

Aysgarth
National Park Centre *tel* (0969) 663424 ♨

Beningborough
Beningborough Hall *tel* (0904) 470666 ♨ *(NT)*

Brimham
Brimham Rocks *tel* (0423) 780688 ♨ *(NT)*

Coxwold
Byland Abbey *tel* (03476) 614

Elvington
Yorkshire Air Museum & Allied Air Forces Memorial *tel* (090485) 595 ♨

Fairburn
Fairburn Ings Nature Reserve *tel* (0767) 680551

Grassington
National Park Centre
tel (0756) 752774 ♨

Harrogate
Harlow Carr Botanical Gardens
tel (0423) 565418
The Royal Pump Room Museum
tel (0423) 503340

Hawes
Dales Countryside Museum *tel* (0969) 667450 ♨

Kirby Misperton
Flamingo Land Zoo & Family Funpark
tel (065386) 287 ♨

Kirkham
Kirkham Priory *tel* (065381) 768

Malham
Yorkshire Dales National Park Centre
tel (0729) 830363 ♨

Malton
Castle Howard *tel* (065384) 333 ♨
Eden Camp Modern History Theme Museum
tel (0653) 697777

Masham
Theakston Brewery Visitor Centre
tel (0765) 689057 ♨

North Stainley
Lightwater Valley Theme Park
tel (0765) 635368 & 635321 ♨

Nunnington
Nunnington Hall *tel* (04395) 283 ♨ *(NT)*

Rievaulx
Rievaulx Terrace *tel* (04396) 340 ♨ *(NT)*

Ripon
Fountains Abbey & Studley Royal
tel (0765) 620333 *(NT)*

Whitby
Whitby Museum *tel* (0947) 602908

York
City Art Gallery *tel* (0904) 623839
Fairfax House *tel* (0904) 655543
Guildhall *tel* (0904) 613161
Jorvik Viking Centre *tel* (0904) 643211
Merchant Adventurers' Hall *tel* (0904) 654818
Museum of Automata *tel* (0904) 655550
National Railway Museum *tel* (0904) 621261
Rail Riders World *tel* (0904) 630169
The Bar Convent *tel* (0904) 643238 ♨
Yorkshire Museum & Gardens *tel* (0904) 629745

NORTHAMPTONSHIRE

Canons Ashby
Canons Ashby House *tel* (0327) 860044 ♨ *(NT)*

Holdenby
Holdenby House Gardens *tel* (0604) 770074

Kettering
Alfred East Gallery *tel* (0536) 410333

NORTHUMBERLAND

Bamburgh
Grace Darling Museum *tel* (0665) 720037 ♨

Cambo
Wallington House Garden & Grounds
tel (067074) 283 ♨ *(NT)*

Corbridge
Corbridge Roman Site *tel* (0434) 632349

Ford
Lady Waterford Hall *tel* (089082) 224 ⚜

Mickley
Cherryburn *tel* (0661) 843276 ⚜ *(NT)*

Rothbury
Cragside House & Country Park & Garden
tel (0669) 20333 ⚜ *(NT)*

Walwick
Chesters Roman Fort & Museum
tel (0434) 681379

NOTTINGHAMSHIRE

Farnsfield
White Post Modern Farm Centre
tel (0623) 882977 & 882026

Mansfield
Museum & Art Gallery *tel* (0623) 663088

Newark-on-Trent
Newark Air Museum *tel* (0636) 707170

Nottingham
Canal Museum *tel* (0602) 598835
Castle Museum *tel* (0602) 483504
Industrial Museum *tel* (0602) 284602
The Lace Hall *tel* (0602) 484221
The Tales Of Robin Hood
tel (0602) 483284

OXFORDSHIRE

Banbury
Banbury Museum *tel* (0295) 259855

Burford
Cotswold Wildlife Park *tel* (0993) 823006

Didcot
Didcot Railway Centre *tel* (0235) 817200

Ipsden
Wellplace Bird Farm *tel* (0491) 680473

Oxford
Ashmolean Museum of Art & Archaeology
tel (0865) 278000
The Oxford Story *tel* (0865) 728822

SHROPSHIRE

Acton Burnell
Acton Burnell Castle

Atcham
Attingham Park *tel* (074377) 203 ⚜ *(NT)*

Bridgnorth
Midland Motor Museum *tel* (0746) 761761
Severn Valley Railway *tel* (0299) 403816 ⚜

Burford
Burford House Gardens *tel* (0584) 810777 ⚜

Moreton Corbet
Castle

Much Wenlock
Much Wenlock Museum *tel* (0952) 727773 ⚜

Quatt
Dudmaston *tel* (0746) 780866 ⚜ *(NT)*

Wroxeter
Roman Town *tel* (0743) 761330

SOMERSET

Ilminster
Barrington Court Gardens *tel* (0985) 847777
⚜ *(NT)*

Montacute
Montacute House Garden *tel* (0935) 823289 *(NT)*

Sparkford
Haynes Sparkford Motor Museum
tel (0963) 40804

Yeovilton
Fleet Air Arm Museum *tel* (0935) 840565

SOUTH YORKSHIRE

Barnsley
Monk Bretton Priory *tel* (0226) 204089

Doncaster
Doncaster Museum & Art Gallery
tel (0302) 734293

Rotherham
Art Gallery *tel* (0709) 382121 *ext* 3628/3635

Sheffield
Shepherd Wheel *tel* (0742) 367731

STAFFORDSHIRE

Alton
Alton Towers *tel* (0538) 702200 ⚜

⚜ *Seasonal Opening*
(NT) National Trust

Drayton Manor Park & Zoo *tel* (0827) 287979 ᧒

Lichfield
Lichfield Heritage Exhibition & Treasury
tel (0543) 256611

Moseley
Moseley Old Hall *tel* (0902) 782808 ᧒ *(NT)*

Rugeley
Wolseley Garden Park
tel (0889) 574766 & 574888

Shugborough
Shugborough Hall & Staffordshire County
Museum *tel* (0889) 881388 ᧒ *(NT)*

Stoke-On-Trent
City Museum & Art Gallery *tel* (0782) 202173
Wedgwood Visitor Centre
tel (0782) 204141 & 204218

Whittington
Staffordshire Regiment Museum, Whittington
Barracks *tel* 021-311 3420 & 3229

SUFFOLK

Bungay
The Otter Trust *tel* (0986) 893470 ᧒

Bury St Edmunds
The Clock Museum *tel* (0284) 757072 (Mon-Fri)
& 757076

Cavendish
Sue Ryder Foundation Museum
tel (0787) 280252

Flixton
Norfolk & Suffolk Aviation Museum
tel (0508) 480778 ᧒

Horringer
Ickworth *tel* (028488) 270 ᧒ *(NT)*

Leiston
Leiston Abbey

Lindsey
St James' Chapel

Long Melford
Melford Hall *tel* (0787) 880286 ᧒ *(NT)*

Lowestoft
Maritime Museum *tel* (0502) 561963 ᧒
Pleasurewood Hills American Theme Park
tel (0502) 513626 ᧒

Newmarket
National Horseracing Museum *tel* (0638) 667333 ᧒

Saxmundham
Bruisyard Winery, Vineyard, Herb & Water
Garden *tel* (072875) 281 ᧒

Southwold
Southwold Museum *tel* (0502) 722375 ᧒

Suffolk Wildlife & Rare Breeds Park
tel (0502) 740291 ᧒

SURREY

Ash Vale
RAMC Historical Museum
tel (0252) 24431 *ext* Keogh 5212

Camberley
Surrey Heath Museum *tel* (0276) 686252

Charlwood
Gatwick Zoo & Aviaries *tel* (0293) 862312

Compton
Watts Picture Gallery *tel* (0483) 810235

East Clandon
Hatchlands *tel* (0483) 222787 ᧒ *(NT)*

Esher
Claremont Landscaped Garden
tel (0372) 469930 *(NT)*

Farnham
Birdworld & Underwaterworld
tel (0420) 22140

Great Bookham
Polesden Lacey *tel* (0372) 458203 *(NT)*

Hascombe
Winkworth Arboretum *tel* (0486) 32477 *(NT)*

West Clandon
Clandon Park *tel* (0483) 222482 ᧒ *(NT)*

Wisley
Wisley Gardens *tel* (0483) 224234

TYNE AND WEAR

Newcastle upon Tyne
Museum of Antiquities *tel* 091-222 7844
Museum of Science & Engineering
tel 091-232 6789

Rowlands Gill
Gibside Chapel & Avenue
tel (0207) 542255 ᧒ *(NT)*

South Shields
South Shields Museum & Art Gallery
tel 091-456 8740

Sunderland
Monkwearmouth Station Museum
tel 091-567 7075
Museum & Art Gallery *tel* 091-514 1235

Washington
Old Hall *tel* 091-416 6879 ⋇ *(NT)*
The Wildfowl & Wetlands Trust
tel 091-416 5454

WARWICKSHIRE

Baddesley Clinton
Baddesley Clinton House
tel (0564) 783294 ⋇ *(NT)*

Charlecote
Charlecote Park *tel* (0789) 470277 ⋇ *(NT)*

Coughton
Coughton Court *tel* (0789) 762435 ⋇ *(NT)*

Packwood House *tel* (0564) 782024 ⋇ *(NT)*

Royal Leamington Spa
Warwick District Council Art Gallery & Museum
tel (0926) 426559

Stratford-Upon-Avon
World Of Shakespeare *tel* (0789) 269190

Twycross
Twycross Zoo Park *tel* (0827) 880250

Upton House *tel* (029587) 266 ⋇ *(NT)*

WEST MIDLANDS

Birmingham
Birmingham Botanical Gardens & Glasshouses
tel 021-454 1860
Birmingham Nature Centre *tel* 021-472 7775
Museum of Science & Industry *tel* 021-236 1022
The Patrick Collection *tel* 021-459 9111

Bournville
Cadbury World *tel* 021-433 4334

⋇ *Seasonal Opening*
(NT) National Trust

Coventry
Herbert Art Gallery *tel* (0203) 832381
Lunt Roman Fort *tel* (0203) 832381 ⚲
Museum of British Road Transport
tel (0203) 832425

Dudley
Dudley Zoo & Castle *tel* (0384) 252401

Ryton-on-Dunsmore
Ryton Gardens *tel* (0203) 303517

Walsall
Walsall Leather Centre Museum
tel (0922) 721153

Wolverhampton
Wightwick Manor *tel* (0902) 761108 ⚲ *(NT)*

WEST SUSSEX

Amberley
Amberley Chalk Pits Museum
tel (0798) 831370 ⚲

Ardingly
Wakehurst Place Garden *tel* (0444) 892701 *(NT)*

Arundel
Wildfowl & Wetlands Trust *tel* (0903) 883355

Ashington
Holly Gate Cactus Garden *tel* (0903) 892930

Bignor
Bignor Roman Villa & Museum *tel* (07987) 259 ⚲

Chichester
Guildhall Museum *tel* (0243) 784683 ⚲
Mechanical Music & Doll Collection
tel (0243) 785421

East Grinstead
Standen *tel* (0342) 323029 ⚲ *(NT)*

Fishbourne
Roman Palace *tel* (0243) 785859

Fontwell
Denmans Garden *tel* (0243) 542808 ⚲

Goodwood
Goodwood House *tel* (0243) 774107 ⚲

Handcross
Nymans Garden
tel (0444) 400321 & 400002 ⚲ *(NT)*

Highdown *tel* (0903) 501054

Petworth
Petworth House *tel* (0798) 42207 ⚲ *(NT)*

Tangmere
Tangmere Military Aviation Museum Trust
tel (0243) 775223 ⚲

Worthing
Worthing Museum & Art Gallery
tel (0903) 239999 *ext* 2528

WEST YORKSHIRE

Bradford
Cartwright Hall Art Gallery *tel* (0274) 493313
Colour Museum *tel* (0274) 390955
Industrial Museum *tel* (0274) 631756
National Museum of Photography,
Film & Television *tel* (0274) 727488

Halifax
Calderdale Industrial Museum
tel (0422) 358087
Piece Hall *tel* (0422) 358087

Harewood
Harewood House & Bird Garden
tel (0532) 886225 ⚲

Haworth
Keighley & Worth Valley Railway & Museum
tel (0535) 645214

Holmfirth
Holmfirth Postcard Museum
tel (0484) 682231

Huddersfield
Art Gallery *tel* (0484) 513808 *ext* 216
Tolson Memorial Museum *tel* (0484) 530591

Keighley
East Riddlesden Hall
tel (0535) 607075 ⚲ *(NT)*

Leeds
Armley Mills Museum *tel* (0532) 637861
Thwaite Mills *tel* (0532) 496453

Middlestown
The Yorkshire Mining Museum
tel (0924) 848806

Nostell Priory *tel* (0924) 863892 ⚲ *(NT)*

Pontefract
Pontefract Museum *tel* (0977) 797289

Shipley
Commonwealth Institute Northern Regional Centre *tel* (0274) 530251

WIGHT, ISLE OF

Arreton
Robin Hill Adventure Park
tel (0983) 527352 & 528029 ※

Brading
Animal World of Natural History
tel (0983) 407286
Lilliput Doll & Toy Museum *tel* (0983) 407231

East Cowes
Barton Manor Vineyard & Gardens
tel (0983) 292835 ※

Godshill
Old Smithy Tourist Centre
tel (0983) 840242 & 840364 ※

WILTSHIRE

Avebury
Great Barn Museum of Wiltshire Life
tel (06723) 555

Bradford On Avon
The Crocker Collection *tel* (02216) 4783 ※
Tithe Barn

Corsham
Corsham Court *tel* (0249) 712214 ※

Great Bedwyn
Bedwyn Stone Museum *tel* (0672) 870043

Lacock
Lacock Abbey *tel* (024973) 227 ※ *(NT)*

Lydiard House & Park *tel* (0793) 770401

Middle Woodford
Heale Gardens & Plant Centre
tel (072273) 504

Salisbury
Museum of the Duke of Edinburgh's Royal Regiment *tel* (0722) 414536

Stourhead
Stourhead House & Garden *tel* (0747) 840348 *(NT)*

Stourton
Stourton House Garden *tel* (0747) 840417 ※

Teffont Magna
Farmer Giles Farmstead *tel* (0722) 716338 ※

Woodhenge

CHANNEL ISLANDS

GUERNSEY

Catel
Le Friquet Butterfly Centre *tel* (0481) 54378 ※

St Andrew
German Military Underground Hospital & Ammunition Store *tel* (0481) 39100

St Peter Port
Guernsey Museum & Art Gallery
tel (0481) 726518

JERSEY

St Lawrence
German Underground Hospital
tel (0534) 863442 ※

St Peter
Jersey Motor Museum *tel* (0534) 482966 ※

Trinity
Jersey Zoological Park *tel* (0534) 864666

ISLE OF MAN

Ballaugh
Curraghs Wild Life Park
tel (062489) 7323 ※

Douglas
Manx Museum *tel* (0624) 675522

NORTHERN IRELAND

ANTRIM

Antrim
Shane's Castle *tel* (08494) 63380 & 28216 ※

Carrickfergus
Town Walls

Giant's Causeway
Giant's Causeway Centre *tel* (02657) 31855

Portballintrae
Dunluce Castle *tel* (02657) 31938

※ *Seasonal Opening*
(NT) National Trust

ARMAGH

Armagh
Armagh Friary

Moy
Argory *tel* (08687) 84753 🦽 *(NT)*

Portadown
Ardress House *tel* (0762) 851236 🦽 *(NT)*

BELFAST

Belfast Castle *tel* (0232) 776925
Belfast Zoological Gardens *tel* (0232) 776277

DOWN

Ballywalter
Grey Abbey

Downpatrick
Inch Abbey

Holywood
Ulster Folk and Transport Museum
tel (0232) 428428

Newtownards
Mount Stewart House, Garden & Temple of the
Winds *tel* (024774) 387 🦽 *(NT)*

Portaferry
Northern Ireland Aquarium *tel* (02477) 28062

Saintfield
Rowallane Garden *tel* (0238) 510131 *(NT)*

Strangford
Castle Ward *tel* (039686) 204 🦽 *(NT)*

FERMANAGH

Belleek
Belleek Pottery *tel* (036565) 501

Enniskillen
Castle Coole *tel* (0365) 322690 🦽 *(NT)*
Florence Court *tel* (036582) 249 🦽 *(NT)*

LONDONDERRY

Cookstown
Springhill *tel* (0648) 748210 🦽 *(NT)*

TYRONE

Ballygawley
US Grant Ancestral Homestead & Visitor Centre
tel (066252) 7133 🦽

SCOTLAND

BORDERS

Duns
Jim Clark Room *tel* (0361) 82600 *ext* 36 🦽

Kelso
Floors Castle *tel* (0573) 2333 🦽
Kelso Abbey *tel* 031-244 3101

Melrose
Melrose Abbey & Abbey Museum
tel 031-244 3101

Selkirk
Bowhill House & Country Park
tel (0750) 20732 🦽

CENTRAL

Bannockburn
Bannockburn Heritage Centre *tel* (0786) 812664

Blair Drummond
Blair Drummond Safari & Leisure Park
tel (0786) 841456 🦽

Callander
Rob Roy and Trossachs Visitor Centre
tel (0877) 30342

Doune
Doune Motor Museum *tel* (0786) 841203 🦽

Stirling
Smith Art Gallery & Museum *tel* (0786) 71917

DUMFRIES & GALLOWAY

Caerlaverock
Caerlaverock Castle *tel* 031-244 3101

Castle Douglas
Threave Garden *tel* (0556) 2575

Creetown
Creetown Gem Rock Museum
tel (067182) 357 & 554

Dumfries
Robert Burns Centre *tel* (0387) 64808

Glenluce
Glenluce Abbey *tel* 031-244 3101

New Abbey
Sweetheart Abbey *tel* 031-244 3101

Port Logan
Logan Botanic Garden *tel* (0776) 86231 ⚘

Ruthwell
Savings Bank Museum *tel* (038787) 640

Stranraer
Castle Kennedy Gardens *tel* (0776) 2024 ⚘

Thornhill
Drumlanrig Castle
tel (0848) 31682 & 30248 ⚘

Wanlockhead
Museum of Lead Mining
tel (0659) 74387 ⚘

Whithorn
Whithorn Priory *tel* 031-244 3101

FIFE

Anstruther
Scottish Fisheries Museum *tel* (0333) 310628

Ceres
Fife Folk Museum
tel (033482) 380 (curator's home) ⚘

Cupar
The Scottish Deer Centre *tel* (033781) 391 ⚘

St Andrews
British Golf Museum *tel* (0334) 78880

GRAMPIAN

Aberdeen
Aberdeen Art Gallery *tel* (0224) 646333
Cruickshank Botanic Garden *tel* (0224) 272704
Satrosphere ('Hands-On' Science & Technology
Exhibition Centre) *tel* (0224) 213232

Brodie Castle *tel* (03094) 371 ⚘

Buckie
Buckie Museum & Peter Anson Gallery
tel (0309) 73701

Dufftown
Dufftown Museum *tel* (0309) 73701 ⚘

Forres
Dallas Dhu Distillery *tel* 031-244 3101 ⚘

Kildrummy
Kildrummy Castle *tel* 031-244 3101

Maryculter
Storybook Glen *tel* (0224) 732941

Methlick
Haddo House *tel* (06515) 440

Pitmedden
Pitmedden Garden *tel* (06513) 2352

Tolquhon Castle *tel* 031-244 3101

Spey Bay
Tugnet Ice House *tel* (0309) 73701 ⚘

Tomintoul
Tomintoul Museum *tel* (0309) 73701 ⚘

HIGHLAND

Alness
Dalmore Farm Centre *tel* (0349) 883978

Armadale
Clan Donald Centre *tel* (04714) 305 & 227 ⚘

Aviemore
Strathspey Railway *tel* (0479) 810725 ⚘

Culloden Moor
Culloden Battlefield *tel* (0463) 790607

Drumnadrochit
Official Loch Ness Monster Exhibition
tel (04562) 573 & 218

Gairloch
Gairloch Heritage Museum *tel* (044583) 243 ⚘

Glenfinnan
Jacobite Monument *tel* (039783) 250 ⚘

Newtonmore
Clan Macpherson House & Museum
tel (05403) 332 ⚘

Poolewe
Inverewe Garden *tel* (044586) 200

Strathpeffer
Strathpeffer Station Visitor Centre
tel (046373) 505 ⚘

Wick
Caithness Glass Factory & Visitor Centre
tel (0955) 2286

LOTHIAN

Dalkeith
Edinburgh Butterfly & Insect World
tel 031-663 4932 ⚘

⚘ *Seasonal Opening*
(NT) National Trust

Dirleton
Dirleton Castle *tel* 031-244 3101

East Fortune
Museum of Flight *tel* (0620) 88308 &
031-225 7534 ❧

Edinburgh
City Art Centre *tel* 031-225 2424
Edinburgh Castle *tel* 031-244 3101
Edinburgh Zoo *tel* 031-334 9171
National Gallery of Scotland *tel* 031-556 8921
Royal Botanic Garden *tel* 031-552 7171
Royal Museum of Scotland (Chambers St)
tel 031-225 7534
Royal Museum of Scotland (Queen St)
tel 031-225 7534
Royal Observatory Visitor Centre
tel 031-668 8405
Scottish National Gallery of Modern Art
tel 031-556 8921
Scottish National Portrait Gallery
tel 031-556 8921
Scottish United Services Museum
tel 031-225 7534
West Register House *tel* 031-556 6585

Gogar
Suntrap Garden & Advice Centre
tel 031-339 7283 & (0506) 854387

Ingliston
Scottish Agricultural Museum
tel 031-225 7534 *ext* 313 ❧

Penicuik
Edinburgh Crystal Visitor Centre
tel (0968) 75128

South Queensferry
Dalmeny House *tel* 031-331 1888 ❧

SHETLAND

Lerwick
Shetland Museum *tel* (0595) 5057

STRATHCLYDE

Alloway
Burns' Cottage *tel* (0292) 41215
Land O'Burns Centre *tel* (0292) 43700

Barcaldine
Sea Life Centre *tel* (0631) 72386 ❧

Bearsden
Roman Bath-House *tel* 031-244 3101

Biggar
Gladstone Court Museum *tel* (0899) 21050 ❧
Moat Park Heritage Centre *tel* (0899) 21050

Coatbridge
Summerlee Heritage Trust *tel* (0236) 31261

Craignure
Mull & West Highland Narrow Gauge Railway
tel (06802) 494 (in season) and
(0680) 300389 ❧

Culzean
Culzean Castle *tel* (06556) 274 ❧
Culzean Country Park *tel* (06556) 269

Glasgow
Burrell Collection *tel* 041-649 7151
Glasgow Art Gallery & Museum
tel 041-357 3929
Greenbank Garden *tel* 041-639 3281
McLellan Galleries *tel* 041-331 1854
Museum of Transport *tel* 041-357 3929
People's Palace *tel* 041-554 0223
Rouken Glen Park *tel* 041-638 1101
University of Glasgow Visitor Centre
tel 041-330 5511

Kilmarnock
Dick Institute *tel* (0563) 26401

Kirkoswald
Souter Johnnie's Cottage *tel* (06556) 603 or 274

Largs
Kelburn Country Centre *tel* (0475) 568685

Lochwinnoch
Lochwinnoch Community Museum
tel (0505) 842615

Maybole
Crossraguel Abbey *tel* 031-244 3101

Millport
Museum of the Cumbraes *tel* (0475) 530741 ❧

Oban
Oban Glassworks *tel* (0631) 63386

Old Dailly
Bargany Gardens *tel* (046587) 227 or 249 ❧

Port Glasgow
Newark Castle *tel* 031-244 3101 ❧

Rothesay
Ardencraig *tel* (0700) 504225
Bute Museum *tel* (0700) 502248

Saltcocks
North Ayrshire Museum *tel* (0294) 64174

Uddingston
Glasgow Zoo *tel* 041-771 1185

TAYSIDE

Blair Atholl
Atholl Country Collection *tel* (079681) 232 ✺

Bruar
Clan Donnachaidh (Robertson) Museum
tel (0796) 483264 ✺

Comrie
Scottish Tartans Museum *tel* (0764) 70779

Dundee
McManus Galleries Museum
tel (0382) 23141 *ext* 65136

Edzell
Edzell Castle *tel* 031-244 3101

Glamis
Angus Folk Museum *tel* (030784) 288 ✺

Kinross
Kinross House Gardens *tel* (0577) 63467 ✺

Perth
Caithness Glass Visitor Centre *tel* (0738) 37373

Pitlochry
Faskally *tel* (03502) 284 ✺

Queen's View
Queen's View Visitor Centre *tel* (03502) 284 ✺

Scone
Scone Palace *tel* (0738) 52300 ✺

WALES

CLWYD

Cerrigydrudion
Llyn Brenig Information Centre *tel* (049082) 463

Wrexham
The Bersham Industrial Heritage Centre
tel (0978) 261529
Erddig *tel* (0978) 355314 ✺ *(NT)*

DYFED

Aberystwyth
National Library of Wales *tel* (0970) 623816

Kidwelly
Kidwelly Industrial Museum *tel* (0554) 891078 ✺

Llanycefn
Penrhos Cottage *tel* (0437) 731328 ✺

Narberth
Oakwood Adventure & Leisure Park
tel (0834) 891376 ✺

Picton Castle
Graham Sutherland Gallery *tel* (0437) 751296 ✺

Ponterwyd
Bwlch Nant-Yr-Arian Forest Visitor Centre
tel (09743) 404 ✺

St Florence
Manor House Wildlife & Leisure Park
tel (0646) 651201 ✺

GWENT

Caerleon
Roman Legionary Museum *tel* (0633) 423134

GWYNEDD

Bangor
Penrhyn Castle *tel* (0248) 353084 ✺ *(NT)*

Betws-Y-Coed
Conwy Valley Railway Museum
tel (0690) 710568 ✺

Blaenau Ffestiniog
Gloddfa Ganol Slate Mine
tel (0766) 830664 ✺

Brynsiencyn
Anglesey Sea Zoo *tel* (0248) 430411

Coed-Y-Brenin
Coed-Y-Brenin Forest Park & Visitor Centre
tel (0341) 422289 ✺

Dinas Mawddwy
Meirion Mill *tel* (06504) 311 ✺

Fairbourne
Fairbourne Railway *tel* (0341) 250362 ✺

✺ *Seasonal Opening*
(NT) National Trust

Llanbedr
Maes Arto Village *tel* (034123) 467 ⚥

Llanberis
Welsh Slate Museum *tel* (0286) 870630 ⚥

Llanystumdwy
Lloyd George Memorial Museum & Highgate Victorian Cottage *tel* (0766) 522071

Plas Newydd *tel* (0248) 714795 ⚥ *(NT)*

Porthmadog
Ffestiniog Railway
tel (0766) 512340 & 831654 ⚥
Ffestiniog Railway Museum
tel (0766) 512340 ⚥

Tal-y-Cafn
Bodnant Garden *tel* (0492) 650460 ⚥

Tywyn
Talyllyn Railway *tel* (0654) 710472 ⚥

MID GLAMORGAN

Merthyr Tydfil
Brecon Mountain Railway *tel* (0685) 384854
Cyfartha Castle Museum & Art Gallery
tel (0685) 723112

Trehafod
Rhondda Heritage Park *tel* (0443) 682036

POWYS

Brecon
The South Wales Borders (24th Regiment) Museum *tel* (0874) 623111 *ext* 2310

Llanfair Caereinion
Welshpool & Llanfair Light (Steam) Railway
tel (0938) 810441 ⚥

Machynlleth
Centre for Alternative Technology
tel (0654) 702400

SOUTH GLAMORGAN

Barry
Welsh Hawking Centre *tel* (0446) 734687

Cardiff
National Museum of Wales (Main Building)
tel (0222) 397951
Techniquest *tel* (0222) 460211
Welsh Industrial & Maritime Museum
tel (0222) 481919

Penarth
Cosmeston Medieval Village
tel (0222) 708686

WEST GLAMORGAN

Cilfrew
Penscynor Wildlife Park *tel* (0639) 642189

Crynant
Cefn Coed Colliery Museum
tel (0639) 750556

Cynonville
Welsh Miners Museum & Afan Argoed Country Park *tel* (0639) 850564 & 850875

Swansea
Swansea Maritime & Industrial Museum Service
tel (0792) 650351

PICNIC SITES

The sites listed below have toilet facilities for the disabled. The sheet number for the relevant Ordnance Survey 1¹/₄″ to 1 mile map is quoted together with the National Grid reference.

ENGLAND

Cambridgeshire

Brandon Creek (A10)

2¹/₂m NE of Littleport Bridge on A10. *(OS143 TL608918)*. Signposted in advance and at entrance. 4 acres, landscaped ground sloping to River Ouse. Furniture.

Cheshire

Hapsford (M56/A5117)

On A5117, near junction with the M56. *(OS117 SJ465745)*. Signposted in advance and at entrance. 2 acres. Useful, utilitarian stopping place near motorway without services. Furniture.

Hartford Picnic Site (A556)

Northwich bypass, 1¹/₂m W of junction with A533. *(OS118 SJ63873)*. 1 acre, useful utilitarian site beside a busy road. Furniture.

Cumbria

Edmond Castle (Off A69)

Midway between Carlisle and Brampton. *(OS86 NY502583)*. 1¹/₂ acre transit area in pleasant farmland. Furniture.

Greenodd Picnic Area (A590)

1m S of Greenodd. *(OS96 SD315816)*. Signposted in advance and at entrance. ¹/₂ acre flat grassland at mouth of estuary amidst undulating countryside of woods and fields. Fishing. Furniture.

White Moss Common (A591)

Old Quarry Car Park 1¹/₂m from Grasmere. *(OS90 NY348066)*. Signposted at entrance. A defunct quarry attractively landscaped and giving access to common land, a conservation area. River fishing may be arranged. Drinking water available.

Derbyshire

Black Rocks (Off B5036)

1m S of Cromford, E of B5035. *(OS119 SK291557)*. Signposted in advance and at entrance. 5 acres. Drinking water available. Furniture.

Middleton Top (Off B5023)

S of Rise End, W of B5023 via unclassified road under old railway bridge. 1m NW of Wirksworth. *(OS119 SK275551)*. 1 acre. Access to Middleton Top Engine House. Furniture.

Staunton Harrold Reservoir (Off B587)

1m SW Melbourne. W of B587 along Calke Lane *(OS128 SK378244)*. Tree-planted grassed area.

Hereford & Worcester

Goodrich Castle (A40)

Ross to Monmouth road, 3¹/₂m from Ross. *(OS162 SO576197)*. Signposted in advance and at entrance. 6 acres. Near entrance to a ruined castle in woods and farmland. Furniture.

Lancashire

Bull Beck (A683)

3m E of M6 junction 34. *(OS97 SD542649)*. Signposted in advance and at entrance. 1 acre, tree-planted area. Furniture.

Spring Wood (A671)   ¹/₂m from Whalley. *(OS103 SD741361)*. Signposted in advance and at entrance. 1 acre, rising to woodland. Furniture.

Leicestershire

Rutland Water Picnic Sites, Sykes Lane (Off A606)   ¹/₂m W of Empingham. *(OS141 SK936083)*. Signposted in advance and at entrance and from adjoining picnic sites. Close to the shore. Tourist Information Centre, telephone, refreshments, furniture. Parking (fee).

Lincolnshire

Legbourne Picnic Place (A157)   W of Legbourne village. *(OS122 TF359847)*. Signposted in advance and at entrance. Hedged and tree-planted grass area. Furniture.

Willingham Ponds (A631)   2m E of Market Rasen. *(OS113 TF137885)*. Signposted in advance and at entrance. Purpose-built area on the forest edge. Furniture.

Somerset

Cartgate Transit Picnic Site (Junction A3088 and A303)   6m NW Yeovil. *(OS198 ST480190)*. Signposted in advance and at entrance. Good parking area with adjacent grassed picnic area. Furniture.

Staffordshire

Waterhouses (Off A523)   At eastern end of Waterhouses Village. *(OS119 SK086511)*. Signposted in advance and at entrance. 3 acres between village and industrial quarries. Situated on high ground above the A523. Furniture.

Wiltshire

Kingston Langley Transit Picnic Sites   2m N of Chippenham. *(OS173 ST911764)*. Signposted in advance and at entrance. Both sides of carriageway screened from traffic. Landscaped grassed areas.

Yorkshire (North)

Staxton Brow (B1249)   ¹/₂m from Staxton Village. *(OS101 TA009779)*. Signposted in advance and at entrance. Sloping tree-planted grass area adjoining separate car park. Panoramic moorland views. Furniture.

WALES

Clywd

Bod Petrual (B5105)   In Clocaenog Forest 6m E of Cerrigydrudion *(OS116 SJ037512)*. An attractive, quiet area in mixed forest by a small lake. Furniture. Toilet facilities closed in winter.

Llangollen, Llantysilio (B5103)   200yds N of A5. *(OS125 SJ197433)*. Signposted in advance and at entrance. 3 acres, quiet woodland on River Dee. Furniture.

Llyn Brenig (Off B4501)   5m N of Cerrigydrudion. *(OS116 SH967547)*. Signposted in advance and at entrance. Extensive lakeside area with many picnic sites, information centre, tea room and viewpoint. Furniture.

Dyfed

Bwlch Nant-yr-Arian (Rheidol Forest) (A44)   10m E of Aberystwyth. *(OS135 SN718813)*. Signposted in advance and at entrance. 10 acre undulating wooded site. Viewpoint, visitor centre and furniture.

Pontarffinant (River Tywi)
Picnic Site (B3400)

1m E of junction with B4310. *(OS159 SN507201).* Signposted in advance and at entrance. 1 acre. Roadside site overlooking River Tywi. Furniture.

Transit Picnic Site
(A40/A478)

1¹/₂m N of Narberth, junction A478/A40. *(OS158 SN122167).* Signposted in advance and at entrance. Level area. Furniture.

Gwynedd
Tan-y-Coed (A487)

Beside A487, 3³/₄m N of Machynlleth. *(OS124 SH755054).* Signposted in advance and at entrance. 2 acres, elevated ground, well-screened. Furniture. Parking (honesty box).

SCOTLAND

Dumfries and Galloway
Garries Park (A75)

Gatehouse of Fleet. *(OS83 NX599561).* 200yds from car park and Tourist Information Centre. 2 acres. Furniture.

Glenairlie Bridge (A76)

On W side of Bridge, 4¹/₂m SE of Sanquhar. *(OS71 NS835058).* Signposted in advance and at entrance. Attractive riverside environment fenced from road. Furniture.

Un-named (B727)

2¹/₂m SW of Kirkcudbright on the Borgue road. *(OS84 NX657486).* Signposted at entrance. 3 acres grassy area in rocky bay. Furniture.

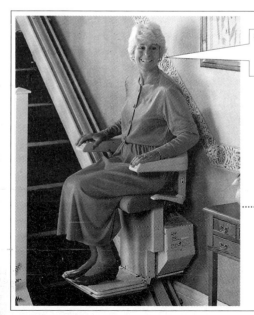

Fife

Edensmuir (B937)

¹/₂m W of Ladybank. *(OS59 NO293094)*. Signposted in advance and at entrance. 3 acres bordered by Cupar Forest. Furniture.

Grampian

Roseisle Picnic Site (B9089)

3m SW of Burghead. *(OS28 NJ105658)*. 30 acres in a pine forest with access to a sandy beach. Furniture. Parking (ticket machine).

Speymouth Forest (A98)

¹/₂m E of Fochabers. *(OS28 NJ358587)*. Signposted in advance and at entrance. On forest road in woodland area. 5 acres. Viewpoint, furniture.

Highland

Daviot Wood (A9)

3m SE of Inverness on the northbound carriageway. *(OS27 NH710414)*. Signposted in advance and at entrance. Attractive and well-maintained site situated in Scots Pine woods, part of the Daviot Wood Information Centre. Viewpoint over the Moray Firth. Furniture.

Invershin (B864)

3m from Invershin Hotel. *(OS27 NH578991)*. Signposted in advance and at entrance. 1¹/₂ acres. Attractive site part-screened at edge of pine forest. Furniture.

North Kessock (A9)

Access from northbound carriageway 200yds from north side of Kessock Bridge. *(OS26 NH655480)*. Signposted in advance and at entrance. Elevated site bounded by shrubs and trees with views over the Beauly Firth. Furniture.

Strathclyde

Duck Bay (A82)

1m N of Balloch. *(OS56 NS373834)*. Signposted in advance and at entrance. 2 acres of grass bordered by trees with view of Loch Lomond. Furniture. Parking by roadside.

Glenfinart Beach Picnic Place

¹/₂m N of Ardentinny off unclassified road to Loch Eck. *(OS56 NS189886)*. Signposted in advance and at entrance. 15 acres backed by forest on a sand and shingle beach. Furniture.

Tayside

Allean-Tummel Forest Park (B8019)

7m N of Pitlochry, ¹/₄m W of Queens View. *(OS43 NN856602)*. Signposted in advance and at entrance. 2 acres, hillside site with part-excavated ring fort. Furniture.

Clova Village (Off B955)

By Clova Hotel. *(OS44 NO327731)*. Small level grass area surrounded by trees. Furniture.

Dalerb (A827)

On N shore at E end of Loch Tay ³/₄m from Kenmore. *(OS52 NS761452)*. Signposted at entrance. Landscaped field with access to rocky shore. Furniture.

Tummel Forest/ Faskally Walk (B8019)

2m N of Pitlochry. *(OS52 NN922592)*. 10 acres in Tummel Forest. Furniture. Parking (ticket machine).

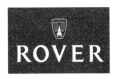

MOTABILITY

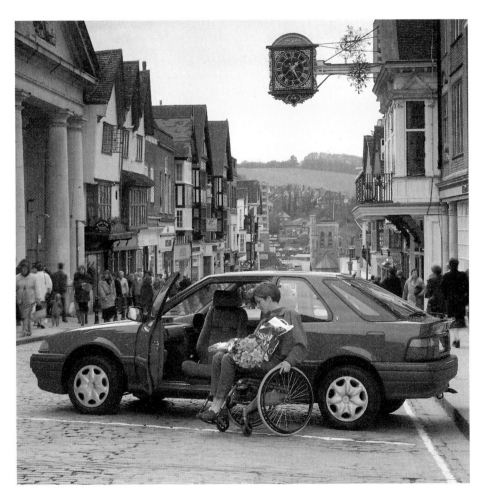

THE ROVER WAY OF LOOKING AT THINGS.

Rover support Motability. Well we would, wouldn't we? We want people to drive Rover cars. But what do we have to offer that's special? First of all, we have one of the widest ranges of cars anywhere.

From the Mini to the Rover 400 Series, we can offer you a car that reflects your personality, your luggage requirements and even the road conditions you're used to.

And at most main Rover Dealers, there is a Motability Adviser to help you get moving as soon as possible.

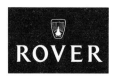

MOTABILITY

Rover cars have a unique blend of build quality, performance and affordable price. The interiors of our cars offer an unusually pleasant and relaxing environment. (We believe you spend more time inside the car than looking at it.) We also have years of experience in conversion.

The Motability Adviser at a Rover Dealer is a specialist trained to understand your individual mobility needs.

Call the Rover Motability helpline on 0345 045310 for details of your nearest Rover Dealer. This service also offers free information and advice on all aspects of Motability and the Rover Cars Mobility scheme.

THE OPTIONS AVAILABLE TO YOU

Motability Contract Hire

This is available over a 3 year period on certain models only. All maintenance and servicing, comprehensive insurance and AA membership are included in the agreement. At the end of the contract period, you return the car to the supplying Dealer and can then open a new contract. This method of payment requires the surrender of your allowance and the payment of an initial rental.

Motability Hire Purchase

With this method you enjoy preferential prices on a new Rover. This option is available over a 4 or 5 year period and enables you to own the vehicle at the end of the contract. This is particularly suitable if complex adaptions are needed.

Rover Cars Mobility Scheme

This is our own scheme, suitable if you are a registered disabled person who is not eligible for a new car through the Motability scheme, or if you prefer not to surrender your allowance. You may also qualify for preferential rates on a new Rover car.

TEST DRIVES AND CONVERSIONS

Test Drives

Whichever Rover you are interested in, try it first before you decide. Ask the Motability Adviser at your local Dealer to arrange a test drive. You will find that typical Rover Motability Advisers are not high-pressure salespeople, but are genuinely helpful and informative.

Conversions

Many adaptions are available. For ease of access, swivel seats can be fitted for the driver and/or front passenger.

Brake, clutch and accelerator can be modified for complete operation by hand, without impairing control of the steering wheel. Other controls can be repositioned where necessary. Hand control systems generally operate using vacuum power from the car to give you a light, positive control requiring minimum effort. Consideration is always given to your own degree of strength for manipulating controls safely.

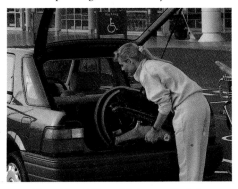

The Motability Adviser will help you choose a car you can get in and out of as easily as possible and will discuss and aim to meet your mobility needs in full. You will above all be treated as an individual.

Once you are a Rover customer, your car will be serviced and maintained with the minimum of fuss and the most advanced technical equipment.

For a free Rover Motability information pack call the Rover Motability helpline on 0345 045310 or complete and post the coupon at the back of this feature.

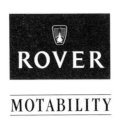

MOTABILITY

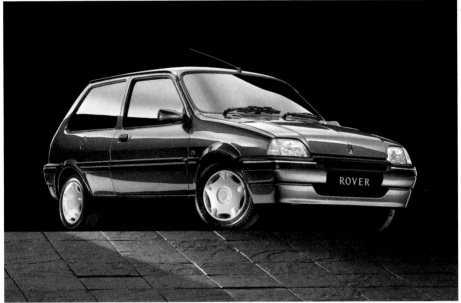

Rover Metro 1.1L

ROVER METRO

The redesigning and re-engineering of the Metro is a famous Rover success story. The new Metro has been called "The best small car in the world," largely because it has the feel of a much bigger car. Powered by the award-winning K-Series engines plus a refined new diesel, the Metro is now available with continuously variable transmission, the leading, smooth automatic transmission of its kind.

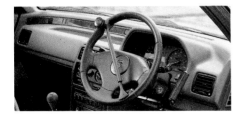

ROVER 200 SERIES

The Rover 200 Series is a hatchback with a good reputation for excellent handling and ride. There are three- and five-door models available with 1.4 or 1.6 litre petrol engines, plus refined and economical diesel versions. The Rover 200 is elegant and thoroughly modern in concept.

ROVER 400 SERIES

The Rover 400 Series is a stylish four-door saloon with a wide range of engines and features on offer. The award-winning 1.4 litre K-Series has excellent performance for its size and at the top of the range 2 litre models are available. The diesel models are becoming increasingly popular. The interior of every model is luxurious and the driving position excellent.

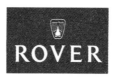

MOTABILITY

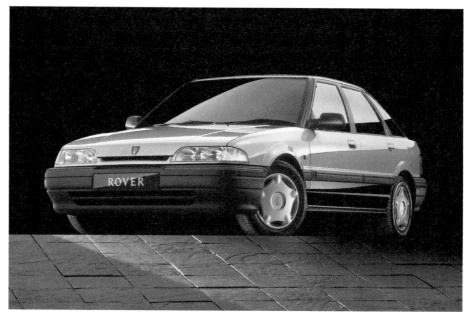

Rover 214 Si

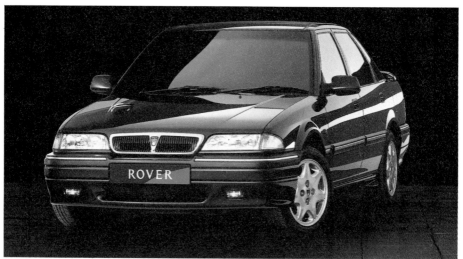

Rover 420 GSi Sport Turbo

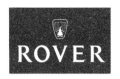

ROVER

MOTABILITY

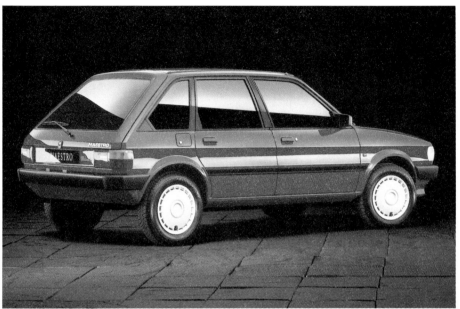

Maestro Clubman D

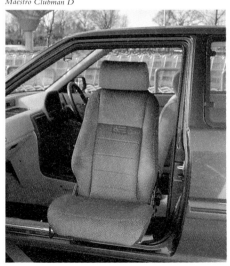

MAESTRO

The ever popular Maestro is a master of two things: space and value for money. This roomy five-door, five-seater hatchback has generous interior space and equipment plus split-folding rear seats. There are two trim levels and engine options, 1.3 petrol and 2.0 litre diesel – the diesel is now turbocharged for better performance and economy and has power steering as an option.

MONTEGO

There are both saloon and estate versions of the accommodating Montego. Generous interiors are complemented by a large load-space and most models, including the estate, have split-folding rear seats. A comfortable driving position and good visibility are also features of this popular, roomy and durable car. Petrol and diesel versions are on offer.

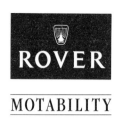

MOTABILITY

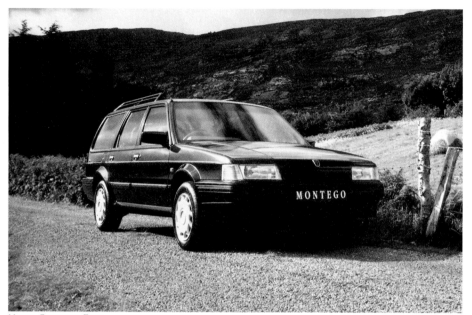

Montego Countryman Estate

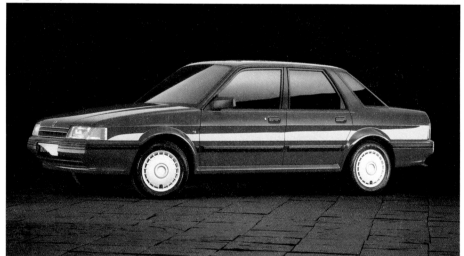

Montego Clubman Diesel

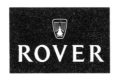

ROVER

MOTABILITY

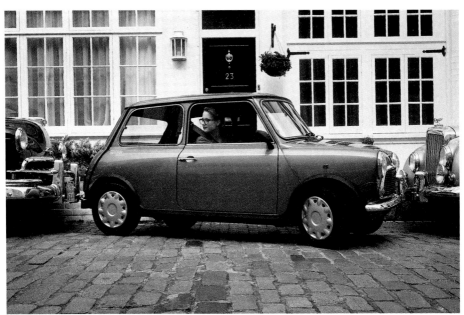

Mini Mayfair

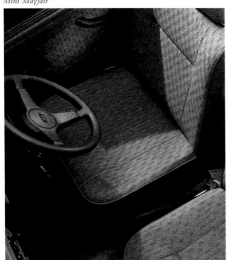

MINI

What can you say about the Mini? For over 30 years it has been a symbol of the sheer joy of driving and is as eager and manoeuvrable as ever. Behind the timeless styling lies a deceptively roomy interior. Today, the Mini is powered by 1.3 litre engines. The Mini offers exceptional value for money and is cheap to maintain. So if you like driving and appreciate its nimble behaviour in town, this British classic is for you.

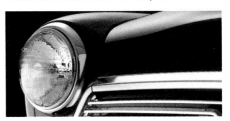

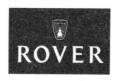

MOTABILITY

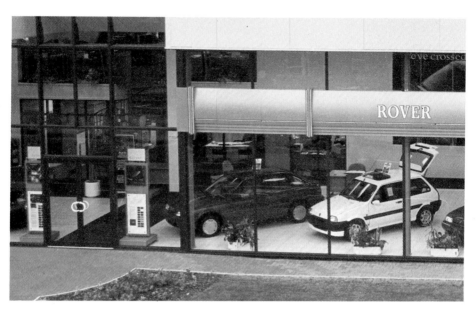

WHAT TO DO NEXT

We hope here to have given you a clear outline of Rover's involvement in Motability and the range of cars available for conversion. For more information, contact your Rover Dealer on the Rover Motability helpline.

For a free Rover Motability information pack, call the helpline on 0345 045310 or complete and post the coupon opposite.

Rover Motability,
FREEPOST, LOL 2105, Dunstable, Beds. LU5 4BR.

MOTABILITY

Please send me details of the Rover Motability programme.

Name _____

Address _____

_____

_____ Postcode _____

Telephone No. _____ Ref: AA/9394

Send to: Rover Motability, FREEPOST, LOL 2105, Dunstable, Beds. LU5 4BR.   No stamp necessary.

ACCOMMODATION

ABOUT THE DIRECTORY

This guide lists Hotels (★s), AA Lodges (⌂), Guesthouses (GH), Farmhouses (FH), Inns (INN), Country House Hotels (⚑♥) and Town and Country Homes (T&C) which provide accommodation suitable for disabled people who are confined to wheelchairs. The information is arranged by county order within country. Many other premises provide facilities for people with greater mobility but these have not been listed. **When making a reservation it is most important that disabled persons inform the receptionist of their disability.**

BASIC REQUIREMENTS

1 Many establishments do not have ground floor bedrooms. For those which do not, a lift, minimum size 3ft 10in deep, 2ft 6in wide, must be available to reach suitable rooms.

2 A maximum of two steps to an entrance. A ramp is acceptable, although in some cases it may be portable.

3 A public or private lavatory must be available, with minimum dimensions of 5ft 4in x 3ft 7in, to enable a wheelchair to be manoeuvred. Intending guests should ensure their room either has a private bathroom/toilet of such dimensions, or is within easy reach of a similarly-sized public lavatory.

4 Entrance doors should be at least 2ft 6in wide, as should doors to bedrooms, bathrooms and public rooms.

5 If the dining room cannot be reached easily then room service must be available.

DIRECTORY ENTRY

County Refers to the administrative or metropolitan county in England, Wales and Ireland or administrative region of Scotland, in which the establishment is situated; it is not necessarily the correct postal address. For places in Scotland, the region is given, followed by the old county in brackets.

Town The town or village in which the establishment is located.

Hotel ★s/⌂/GH/FH/INN/⚑♥/T&C address The name of the establishment and street/road name.

Seasonal opening Establishments are not necessarily open all year and it is advisable to check.

Telephone number for reservations The area code appears in brackets before the telephone number. Unless otherwise shown the code is that of the town under which the establishment is listed.

Classification The Automobile Association's classification of the establishment (*see page 43*).

Entrance Refers to the recommended access to the establishment for disabled persons.

Steps Indicates the number of steps (or ramp) at the recommended entrance. It should be noted that ramps can be of the portable type and have to be requested in advance.

Doors The type of doors to be found at the recommended entrance. If revolving doors are in place, they can be folded back to give a minimum width of 2ft 6in.

Bedrooms The number of bedrooms shown are those that are easily accessible by a wheelchair, on the ground floor. Other bedrooms may be available on a floor served by a suitably sized lift.

Lifts These may assist access to bedrooms and/or public rooms not situated on the ground floor. Minimum dimensions should be 3ft 10in deep by 2ft 6in wide. (See also 'Fire precautions' paragraph).

Toilet information This details establishments providing **suitable** toilet facilities *en suite*. However, it is emphasised that only a limited number may be suitable for disabled people, and in some cases access to public toilets/bathrooms is limited. In establishments where suitable toilets are not provided *en suite*, adequate public toilet and bathroom facilities exist within easy reach of bedrooms.

Room Service This is particularly useful in those establishments where access to the dining room may be difficult. It may not normally be available to the public but can be arranged for disabled people.

Dining room Accessible without difficulty. If the dining room is not accessible, room service should be available, although it may have to be requested in advance and the hours of service may be limited.

Telephone/Intercom This indicates whether there is some form of direct communication between the bedroom and reception.

Guide dogs allowed Notice should be given to the establishment if a guide dog is to accompany the guest as there may be restrictions.

Parking at entrance This indicates that it is possible to stop at the recommended hotel entrance to unload passengers and luggage.

Access to reception Accessible without difficulty.

Access to lounge Accessible without difficulty.

Access to bar Accessible without difficulty.

GH FH INN Guesthouses, Farmhouses and Inns Guesthouses, including small and private hotels and inns, provide comfortable accommodation but without some of the services or facilities available at star-rated hotels. Full details of these are provided in the *AA Inspected Bed and Breakfast in Britain and Ireland,* published annually, and the *AA Members' Handbook* (members only).

T&C Town and Country Homes This classification is applicable only within the Republic of Ireland and is denoted by the symbol T&C. Full details of these are provided in the *AA Members' Handbook Ireland* (members only).

Reservations It is advisable to book early, especially during the holiday season. You should inform the hotel staff at once of any delay or change of plan since you may be held legally responsible for part of the charge if the room booked cannot be re-let.

When making a booking it is **most important** that disabled persons acquaint the establishment concerned with the extent of their disability and obtain confirmation that the facilities are still available as described in the directory. On arrival the reception staff should be advised of the disability so that adequate arrangements can be made in the event of fire or other emergency.

POINTS TO CONSIDER WHEN BOOKING AN HOTEL ROOM

Annexes In some cases suitable bedrooms will be in an annexe and facilities may not be the same as in the main building. Therefore, it is advisable to check the nature of accommodation before making a reservation.

Cheques Are cheques acceptable and how much notice, if any, is required?

Credit cards Some establishments may accept payment by credit cards.

Children Not all hotels accept children; you should check restrictions before making reservations.

Deposits Are you prepared to pay a deposit for short stays, particularly if no advance booking was made? Some hotels now demand full payment for accommodation prior to checking in, particularly for one night stays.

Night porter Probably available in four and five-star hotels.

Fire precautions From our own enquiries every hotel in Great Britain listed in this publication has applied for and not been refused a fire certificate at the time of going to press. It is most important that hotel staff are aware of a disability which might affect an escape in the event of a fire, especially if a lift is grounded during an emergency.

Hygiene Local authorities are responsible for enforcing legislation governing conditions of hygiene in hotels. Our inspectors satisfy themselves that standards are being maintained at an acceptable level.

Prices Please refer to the current *AA Members' Handbook* and *AA Members' Handbook Ireland* (members only); *Hotels and Restaurants in Britain and Ireland* or the *AA Inspected Bed and Breakfast in Britain and Ireland* (both saleable publications) for details.

The hotel industry's voluntary Code of Booking Practice was introduced in June 1977 and revised in 1986. Its prime object is to ensure that the customer is clear about the precise service and facilities he is buying, and what price he will have to pay, before he commits himself to a contractually binding agreement.

Unless provided with written proof of the obligatory charge prior to reaching the property the guest should be handed a card at the time of registration, quoting the total obligatory charge, and details may also be displayed prominently at the reception office. The Tourism (Sleeping Accommodation Price Display) Order 1977 was introduced in February 1978. It compels hotels, motels, guesthouses, inns and self-catering accommodation with four or more letting bedrooms to display in entrance halls the maximum and minimum prices charges for each category of room. This order complements the voluntary Code of Booking Practice.

Every effort is being made by the AA to encourage the use of the voluntary Code in appropriate establishments.

Outside Great Britain other regulations concerning price display may apply.

Meals All hotels with a star classification are expected to serve breakfast, lunch and dinner for residents seven days a week. Meal facilities are increasingly more limited for non-residents especially in lower classified properties. In some parts of the country high tea is served rather than dinner and an element of self-service is increasingly found at certain meals. Non-residents are advised to check in advance that the required meal will be available.

Telephone surcharge A surcharge is sometimes imposed on telephone calls made through the hotel switchboard and guests should check the amount before placing a call.

Complaints These should be taken up with the management at the time. If a personal approach fails, inform the AA as soon as possible so that investigations may be made. State whether your name may be disclosed to the hotel.

Please contact:

Hotel Services Department,
The Automobile Association,
Fanum House,
Basingstoke,
Hants
RG21 2EA.

HOTEL CLASSIFICATION

The star classification of hotels by the AA, in addition to providing an indication of the type of hotel, may be regarded as a universally accepted standard from the simplest to the most luxurious hotel.

AA Travel Lodge ⌂   Bedroom accommodation block, of at least two star standard, all rooms with private facilities. As a general rule restaurant/dining facilities are to be found in the adjacent motorway or roadside restaurant.

★   Hotels generally of small scale with good facilities and furnishings. Adequate bath and lavatory arrangements. Meals are provided for residents but their availability to non-residents may be limited. The AA now accepts private hotels at one and two star level, where the requirements for ready public access and full lunch service may be relaxed.

★★   Hotels offering a higher standard of accommodation and some bedrooms containing a private bathroom/shower-room with lavatory. The AA now accepts private hotels at one and two star level, where the requirements for ready public access and full lunch service may be relaxed.

★★★   Well-appointed hotels with more spacious accommodation with the majority of bedrooms containing a private bathroom/shower-room with lavatory. Fuller meal facilities are provided.

★★★★   Exceptionally well-appointed hotels offering a high standard of comfort and service with bedrooms providing a private bathroom/shower-room with lavatory.

★★★★★ Luxury hotels offering highest international standards.

% The percentage rating is an assessment scheme whereby hotels are awarded a percentage score, within their particular star classification, based on quality.

★ **Red Star** The supreme award used to denote hotels considered to be of outstanding merit within their classification.

🌲 The symbol used to denote an AA Country House hotel where a relaxed informal atmosphere and personal welcome prevail. However, some of the facilities may differ from those found in urban hotels of the same classification.

For more detailed information about our appointed/listed hotels you are advised to refer to the *AA Members' Handbook* and *AA Members' Handbook Ireland* (members only); *Hotels and Restaurants in Britain and Ireland* and the *AA Inspected Bed and Breakfast in Britain and Ireland* (both saleable publications).

The information contained within the guide on accommodation has been supplied by the hotel and guesthouse proprietors, and its accuracy is checked very carefully. However, when making a booking, members should acquaint the establishment concerned with the extent of their disability and obtain confirmation that the facilities available are still as described in the directory to ensure that they are comfortably accommodated. The AA cannot accept any responsibility for omissions and errors, but should members find the facilities at any hotel to be different from those described, please let us know so that we can investigate the matter.

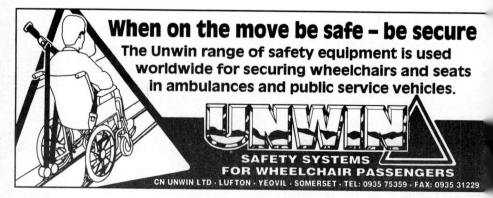

ALPHABETICAL LIST OF ACCOMMODATION BY TOWN

ENGLAND

Abingdon, *Oxfordshire* 76
Acle, *Norfolk* 72
Adlington, *Cheshire* 51
Aldeburgh, *Suffolk* 80
Alfreton, *Derbyshire* 55
Allendale, *Northumberland* 73
Alston, *Cumbria* 53
Alwalton, *Cambridgeshire* 50
Ambleside, *Cumbria* 54
Amesbury, *Wiltshire* 85
Ampfield, *Hampshire* 61
Andover, *Hampshire* 62
Appleby-in-Westmorland,
  Cumbria 54
Ashbourne, *Derbyshire* 55
Ashburton, *Devon* 56
Ashford, *Kent* 65
Aston Clinton,
  Buckinghamshire 50
Aust Motorway Service Area,
  Avon 48
Aylesbury, *Buckinghamshire* 50

Bakewell, *Derbyshire* 56
Baldock, *Hertfordshire* 64
Barnham Broom, *Norfolk* 72
Barnsley, *South Yorkshire* 78
Barnstaple, *Devon* 56
Barton Mills, *Suffolk* 80
Barton Stacey, *Hampshire* 62
Barton-Under-Needwood,
  Staffordshire 79
Basildon, *Essex* 59
Basingstoke, *Hampshire* 62
Bath, *Avon* 48
Batley, *West Yorkshire* 84
Bebington, *Merseyside* 71
Bedford, *Bedfordshire* 48
Beverley, *Humberside* 64
Birdlip, *Gloucestershire* 60
Birmingham, *West Midlands* 82
Blakeney, *Norfolk* 72
Blandford Forum, *Dorset* 58
Blyth, *Nottinghamshire* 75
Bolton, *Great Manchester* 61
Bolton Abbey,
  North Yorkshire 73
Borehamwood, *Hertfordshire* 64
Boroughbridge,
  North Yorkshire 73
Bournemouth, *Dorset* 58
Bourton-on-the-Water,
  Gloucestershire 60
Bracknell, *Berkshire* 49
Bradford, *West Yorkshire* 84
Bramhall, *Cheshire* 51
Brands Hatch, *Kent* 65
Branston, *Lincolnshire* 69
Brentwood, *Essex* 60
Bridgwater, *Somerset* 77
Bridport, *Dorset* 58

Bristol, *Avon* 48
Bromborough, *Merseyside* 71
Bromsgrove,
  Hereford & Worcester 64
Brook, *Hampshire* 62
Bucklow Hill, *Cheshire* 51
Burgh Heath, *Surrey* 81
Burnley, *Lancashire* 66
Bury, *Greater Manchester* 61
Buxton, *Derbyshire* 56

Cambridge, *Cambridgeshire* 50
Carcroft, *South Yorkshire* 78
Carlisle, *Cumbria* 54
Casterton, *Cumbria* 54
Castle Combe, *Wiltshire* 85
Castle Donnington,
  Leicestershire 67
Castletown, *Man, Isle of* 71
Charlecote, *Warwickshire* 82
Cheltenham, *Gloucestershire* 60
Chester, *Cheshire* 51
Chipping Camden,
  Gloucestershire 60
Chorley, *Lancashire* 66
Cirencester, *Gloucestershire* 61
Clayton-Le-Woods, *Lancashire* 66
Clearwell, *Gloucestershire* 61
Colchester, *Essex* 60
Colsterworth, *Lincolnshire* 69
Colyton, *Devon* 56
Coniston, *Cumbria* 54
Cooden Beach, *East Sussex* 59
Copthorne, *West Sussex* 84
Corby, *Northamptonshire* 72
Coventry, *West Midlands* 83
Crewe, *Cheshire* 52
Croydon, *Greater London* 70

Daventry, *Northamptonshire* 72
Dawlish, *Devon* 56
Derby, *Derbyshire* 56
Desborough,
  Northamptonshire 73
Doncaster, *South Yorkshire* 78
Dorking, *Surrey* 81
Dover, *Kent* 65
Droitwich,
  Hereford & Worcester 64
Dudley, *West Midlands* 83
Dulverton, *Somerset* 77
Dunstable, *Bedfordshire* 49
Durham, *Co Durham* 59

Eastbourne, *East Sussex* 59
East Horndon, *Essex* 60
Eastleigh, *Hampshire* 62
Evershot, *Dorset* 58
Exeter, *Devon* 57

Fairford, *Gloucestershire* 61
Falmouth, *Cornwall* 53
Fareham, *Hampshire* 62

Farthing Corner Motorway
  Service Area, *Kent* 65
Felling, *Tyne & Wear* 81
Ferrybridge Service Area,
  West Yorkshire 85
Five Oaks, *West Sussex* 84
Flitwick, *Bedfordshire* 49
Flore, *Northamptonshire* 73
Fontwell, *West Sussex* 84
Forton Motorway Service Area,
  Lancashire 67
Four Marks, *Hampshire* 62
Frankley Motorway Service
  Area, *West Midlands* 83
Frodsham, *Cheshire* 52

Goodwood, *West Sussex* 84
Gordono Motorway Service
  Area, *Avon* 48
Grantham, *Lincolnshire* 69
Gravesend, *Kent* 65
Great Milton, *Oxfordshire* 76
Greenford, *Kent* 70
Guildford, *Surrey* 81

Hadleigh, *Suffolk* 80
Hailsham, *East Sussex* 59
Harewood, *West Yorkshire* 85
Harrogate, *North Yorkshire* 74
Hartlepool, *Cleveland* 53
Hatfield, *Hertfordshire* 64
Haydock, *Merseyside* 71
Haytor, *Devon* 57
Helmsley, *North Yorkshire* 74
Hereford,
  Hereford & Worcester 64
Heston Motorway Service Area,
  Greater London 70
High Wycombe,
  Buckinghamshire 50
Hillingdon, *Greater London* 70
Hilton Park Motorway Service
  Area, *West Midlands* 83
Hockliffe, *Bedfordshire* 49
Holmes Chapel, *Cheshire* 52
Honiley, *Warwickshire* 82
Hook, *Hampshire* 62
Hooton Roberts,
  South Yorkshire 78
Horrabridge, *Devon* 57
Horton, *Dorset* 58
Hull, *Humberside* 65
Hunstanton, *Norfolk* 72

Ilminster, *Somerset* 77
Ingatestone, *Essex* 60
Ipswich, *Suffolk* 80

Keswick, *Cumbria* 54
Kettlewell, *North Yorkshire* 74
Kidderminster,
  Hereford & Worcester 64
King's Lynn, *Norfolk* 72

ALPHABETICAL LIST OF ACCOMMODATION BY TOWN (Continued)

Knutsford, *Cheshire*   52

Lancaster, *Lancashire*   67
Langho, *Lancashire*   67
Leeming Bar,
   North Yorkshire   74
Lee-on-the-Solent,
   Hampshire   63
Leicester, *Leicestershire*   68
Leigh Delamere Motorway
   Service Area, *Wiltshire*   86
Lew, *Oxfordshire*   76
Leyburn, *North Yorkshire*   74
Leyland, *Lancashire*   67
Limpley Stoke, *Avon*   48
Liverpool, *Merseyside*   72
Lolworth, *Cambridgeshire*   50
London (Central), *NW3*   70
London (Central), *SW1*   70
London (Central), *W1*   70
London (Central), *W6*   70
London (Central), *W8*   70
Long Eaton, *Derbyshire*   56
Longhorsley,
   Northamptonshire   73
Long Sutton, *Lincolnshire*   69
Lower Beeding, *West Sussex*   84
Lutterworth, *Leicestershire*   68
Lytham St Annes, *Lancashire*   67

Macclesfield, *Cheshire*   52
Maidstone, *Kent*   66
Manchester,
   Greater Manchester   61
Market Drayton,
   Shropshire   76
Markfield,
   Leicestershire   68
Markham Moor,
   Nottinghamshire   75
Marston Moretaine,
   Bedfordshire   49
Melksham, *Wiltshire*   86
Melton Mowbray,
   Leicestershire   68
Meriden, *West Midlands*   83
Middle Wallop, *Hampshire*   63
Mildenhall, *Suffolk*   80
Milton Keynes,
   Buckinghamshire   50
Minehead, *Somerset*   77
Morcott, *Leicestershire*   68
Morden, *Greater London*   70
Mottram St Andrew,
   Cheshire   52
Mudford, *Somerset*   78

Nantwich, *Cheshire*   52
Newark-on-Trent,
   Nottinghamshire   75
Newbury, *Berkshire*   49
Newby Bridge, *Cumbria*   54
Newcastle Upon Tyne,
   Tyne & Wear   81
Newmarket, *Suffolk*   81

Newquay, *Cornwall*   53
Normanton, *Leicestershire*   68
Northallerton,
   North Yorkshire   74
Northampton,
   Northamptonshire   73
North Waltham, *Hampshire*   63
Norwich, *Norfolk*   72
Nottingham, *Nottinghamshire*   75
Nuneaton, *Warwickshire*   82
Nutfield, *Surrey*   81

Oakham, *Leicestershire*   68
Okehampton, *Devon*   57
Oldbury, *West Midlands*   83
Oswestry, *Shropshire*   76
Oxford, *Oxfordshire*   76

Padworth, *Berkshire*   49
Penrith, *Cumbria*   54
Peterborough,
   Cambridgeshire   50
Pevensey, *East Sussex*   59
Plymouth, *Devon*   57
Podimore, *Somerset*   78
Port Isaac, *Cornwall*   53
Portsmouth, *Hampshire*   63
Preston, *Lancashire*   67

Ravenglass, *Cumbria*   54
Ravenstonedale, *Cumbria*   54
Reading, *Berkshire*   49
Redditch,
   Hereford & Worcester   64
Redruth, *Cornwall*   53
Rochester, *Kent*   66
Rossington, *South Yorkshire*   78
Ross-on-Wye,
   Hereford & Worcester   64
Rotherham, *South Yorkshire*   78
Rousdon, *Devon*   57
Rowsley, *Derbyshire*   56
Rugeley, *Staffordshire*   79
Ruislip, *Greater London*   71
Runcorn, *Cheshire*   52

St Austell, *Cornwall*   53
St Ives, *Cambridgeshire*   51
St Leonards, *Dorset*   59
Salisbury, *Wiltshire*   86
Saltash, *Cornwall*   53
Sampford Peverell, *Devon*   58
Sandbach, *Cheshire*   52
Scotch Corner,
   North Yorkshire   74
Seaton Burn, *Tyne & Wear*   81
Sedgemoor Motorway Service
   Area, *Somerset*   78
Shanklin, *Wight, Isle of*   85
Shap, *Cumbria*   55
Sheffield, *South Yorkshire*   79
Shipbourne, *Kent*   66
Sibson, *Warwickshire*   82
Skipton, *North Yorkshire*   74
Sleaford, *Lincolnshire*   69

Slough, *Berkshire*   50
Solihull, *West Midlands*   84
South Normanton,
   Derbyshire   56
Southport, *Merseyside*   72
Southwaite Motorway Service
   Area, *Cumbria*   55
South Witham, *Lincolnshire*   70
Stamford, *Lincolnshire*   69
Standish, *Greater Manchester*   61
Stockton-on-Tees, *Cleveland*   53
Stoke-on-Trent, *Staffordshire*   80
Stone, *Staffordshire*   80
Stourbridge, *West Midlands*   84
Stowmarket, *Suffolk*   81
Stratford-upon-Avon,
   Warwickshire   82
Sturminster Newton, *Dorset*   58
Sunderland, *Tyne & Wear*   81
Sutton, *Greater London*   71
Sutton Scotney, *Hampshire*   63
Swanage, *Dorset*   59
Swindon, *Wiltshire*   86

Tamworth, *Staffordshire*   80
Taunton Deane Motorway
   Service Area, *Somerset*   78
Telford, *Shropshire*   76
Temple Sowerby, *Cumbria*   55
Tetbury, *Gloucestershire*   61
Thatcham, *Berkshire*   50
Thorne, *South Yorkshire*   79
Thornley, *Co Durham*   59
Thrapston,
   Northamptonshire   73
Thrussington,
   Leicestershire   69
Thurcroft, *South Yorkshire*   79
Thurlaston, *Warwickshire*   82
Tiverton, *Devon*   58
Toddington Motorway Service
   Area, *Bedfordshire*   49
Todwick, *South Yorkshire*   79
Tonbridge, *Kent*   66
Torquay, *Devon*   58
Towcester,
   Northamptonshire   73
Treyarnon Bay, *Cornwall*   53
Tunbridge Wells (Royal),
   Kent   66

Uckfield, *East Sussex*   59
Uttoxeter, *Staffordshire*   80

Wakefield, *West Yorkshire*   85
Walsall, *West Midlands*   84
Waltham Abbey, *Essex*   60
Wareham, *Dorset*   59
Warminster, *Wiltshire*   86
Warrington, *Cheshire*   52
Washington Service Area,
   Tyne & Wear   82
Wateringbury, *Kent*   66
Watermillock, *Cumbria*   55
Wentbridge, *West Yorkshire*   85

ALPHABETICAL LIST OF ACCOMMODATION BY TOWN (Continued)

West Drayton,
  Greater London 71
West Thurrock, *Essex* 60
West Witton, *North Yorkshire* 74
Wetheral, *Cumbria* 55
Wetherby, *West Yorkshire* 85
Wheatley, *Oxfordshire* 76
Whickham, *Tyne & Wear* 82
Whitchurch, *Shropshire* 77
Whitley Bay, *Tyne & Wear* 82
Willerby, *Humberside* 65
Winchester, *Hampshire* 63
Windermere, *Cumbria* 55
Wisbech, *Cambridgeshire* 51
Woolley Edge Motorway Service
  Area, *West Yorkshire* 85
Woolverton, *Avon* 48
Wootton Bassett, *Wiltshire* 86
Worfield, *Shropshire* 77
Worksop, *Nottinghamshire* 76
Worthing, *West Sussex* 84
Wrightington, *Lancashire* 67
Wrotham, *Kent* 66

Yarmouth, Great, *Norfolk* 72
York, *North Yorkshire* 74

CHANNEL ISLANDS

JERSEY
St Helier 86
St Saviour 86

WALES

Abersoch, *Gwynedd* 88

Betws-y-Coed, *Gwynedd* 88
Brecon, *Powys* 89
Bridgend, *Mid Glamorgan* 89
Builth Wells, *Powys* 90

Cardiff, *South Glamorgan* 90
Colwyn Bay, *Clwyd* 87
Criccieth, *Gwynedd* 88
Cross Hands, *Dyfed* 87

Dolgellau, *Gwynedd* 88

Halklyn, *Clwydd* 87

Lamphey, *Dyfed* 87
Llandegai, *Gwynedd* 88
Llandudno, *Gwynedd* 89
Llangammarch Wells, *Powys* 90
Llangefni, *Gwynedd* 89
Llanrhystud, *Dyfed* 88

Merthyr Tydfil,
  Mid Glamorgan 89
Monmouth, *Gwent* 88

Newport, *Gwent* 88
Northop Hall, *Clwyd* 87

Pencoed, *Mid Glamorgan* 89
Porthcawl, *Mid Glamorgan* 89
Port Talbot, *West Glamorgan* 90

Rossett, *Clwyd* 87

St Asaph, *Clwyd* 87
Sarn Park Service Area,
  Mid Glamorgan 89
Swansea, *West Glamorgan* 90

Tintern, *Gwent* 88

Wrexham, *Clwyd* 87

SCOTLAND

Aberdeen, *Grampian* 92
Aberlady, *Highland* 93
Auchterarder, *Tayside* 96
Aviemore *Highland* 92

Banchory, *Grampian* 92
Blairgowrie, *Tayside* 96
Brora, *Highland* 93

Callander, *Central* 91
Carrutherstown,
  Dumfries & Galloway 91
Colvend,
  Dumfries & Galloway 91
Connel, *Strathclyde* 94
Contin, *Highland* 93

Dalwhinnie, *Highland* 93
Denny, *Central* 91
Drymen, *Central* 91
Dumbarton, *Strathclyde* 94
Dundee, *Tayside* 96
Dunfermline, *Fife* 92
Dunkeld, *Tayside* 96
Dyce, *Grampian* 92

Edinburgh, *Lothian* 94
Eriska, *Strathclyde* 94
Erskine, *Strathclyde* 94

Gatehouse of Fleet,
  Dumfries & Galloway 91
Glasgow, *Strathclyde* 94
Gretna (with Gretna Green),
  Dumfries & Galloway 91

Huntly, *Grampian* 92

Inverness, *Highland* 93

Kelso, *Borders* 90
Kinclaven, *Tayside* 96
Kinnesswood, *Tayside* 96
Kinross, *Tayside* 96

Kirkmichael, *Tayside* 96

Largs, *Strathclyde* 95
Lockerbie,
  Dumfries & Galloway 91

Mey, *Highland* 93
Moffat, *Dumfries & Galloway* 91
Montrose, *Tayside* 96
Musselburgh, *Lothian* 94

Oban, *Strathclyde* 95
Onich, *Highland* 93

Perth, *Tayside* 96
Pitlochry, *Tayside* 96

Rhu, *Strathclyde* 95

Sanquhar,
  Dumfries & Galloway 92
Spean Bridge, *Highland* 93
St Andrews, *Fife* 92
St Boswells, *Borders* 90
Stirling, *Central* 91
Strachur, *Strathclyde* 95

Troon, *Strathclyde* 95
Turnberry, *Strathclyde* 95

Uddingston, *Strathclyde* 96

IRELAND

Athlone, *Co Westmeath* 98

Blarney, *Co Cork* 97

Cork, *Co Cork* 97

Dublin, *Co Dublin* 98
Dun Laoghaire, *Co Dublin* 98

Ennis, *Co Clare* 97

Holywood, *Co Down* 98

Kilkenny, *Co Kilkenny* 98
Killarney, *Co Kerry* 98
Kinsale, *Co Cork* 97

Lucan, *Co Dublin* 98

Newmarket-on-Fergus,
  Co Clare 97

Rosslare, *Co Wexford* 98

Shannon, *Co Clare* 97

Tralee, *Co Kerry* 98

Westport, *Co Mayo* 98

ENGLAND

AUST MOTORWAY SERVICE AREA **AVON**
(M4, jct 21) BS12 3BJ
☎ Pilning (0454) 633313
PAVILION LODGE ⌂
Access through main double doors via ramp

BATH Sydney Road BA2 6JF **AVON**
☎ (0225) 444424
BATH SPA ★★★★★ **68%**
Access through side double doors from North Road via ramp

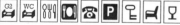

BATH Church Street Bathford BA1 7RR **AVON**
(3m NE on A363) ☎ (0225) 859593
OLD SCHOOL HOUSE GH
Access through main single door from Church Street

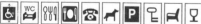

BRISTOL Lower Castle Street **AVON**
BS1 3AD ☎ (0272) 294281
BRISTOL MARRIOTT ★★★★ **59%**
Access through main revolving door from Lower Castle Street

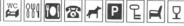

BRISTOL Victoria Street BS1 6HY **AVON**
☎ (0272) 255010
BRISTOL MOAT HOUSE ★★★★ **64%**
Access through main double automatic doors from Victoria Street via ramp

---

BRISTOL College Green BS1 5TA **AVON**
☎ (0272) 255100
SWALLOW ROYAL ★★★★ **73%**
Access through main single, double and revolving doors from College Green via ramp

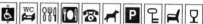

GORDANO MOTORWAY SERVICE **AVON**
AREA (M5) Portbury Bristol BS20 9XG
☎ Pill (027581) 3709 Central Res (0800) 850950
FORTE TRAVELODGE ⌂
Access through main double doors from car park via ramp

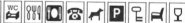

LIMPLEY STOKE Crowe Hill BA3 6HY **AVON**
☎ (0225) 723226
CLIFFE ★★★ **67%**
Access through main double doors from Cliffe Drive via one step

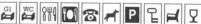

WOOLVERTON BA3 6QS **AVON**
☎ Frome (0373) 830415
WOOLVERTON HOUSE ★★★ **63%**
Access through main double doors from car park via one step. Grab rails around bath only

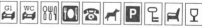

BEDFORD Cardington Road **BEDFORDSHIRE**
Fenlake M44 3SA ☎ (0234) 270044
THE BARNS ★★★ **67%**
Access through main double door via ramp

48

DUNSTABLE* London Road **BEDFORDSHIRE**
LU6 3DX ☎ Luton (0582) 601122
HIGHWAYMAN ★★ **62%**
Access through main double doors from London
Road via ramp

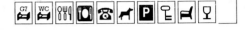

FLITWICK* Church Road **BEDFORDSHIRE**
MK45 1AE ☎ (0525) 712242
FLITWICK MANOR HOTEL ★★★ **74%**
Access through main single door from Church
Road

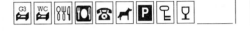

HOCKLIFFE Watling Street **BEDFORDSHIRE**
☎ (0525) 211177 Central Res (0800) 850950
FORTE TRAVELODGE ⌂
Access through main double doors from car park
via ramp

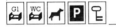

MARSTON MORETAINE **BEDFORDSHIRE**
Beancroft Road Junction MK43 0PQ
☎ Bedford (0234) 766755 Central Res (0800) 850950
FORTE TRAVELODGE ⌂
Access through main double doors from car park
via ramp

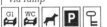

TODDINGTON MOTORWAY **BEDFORDSHIRE**
SERVICE AREA M1 Motorway LU5 6HR
☎ (0525) 875150
GRANADA LODGE ⌂
Access through main double doors from car park
via ramp

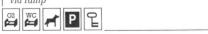

BRACKNELL Maidens Green **BERKSHIRE**
RG12 6LD ☎ (0344) 882284
STIRRUPS COUNTRY HOUSE ★★★ **65%**
Access through side double swing doors from
Bracknell Road via ramp. Grab rails around bath
only

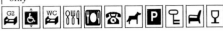

NEWBURY Old Oxford Road **BERKSHIRE**
Donnington RG16 9AG
☎ (0635) 551199
DONNINGTON VALLEY ★★★★ **68%**
Access through automatic main door via ramp

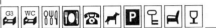

PADWORTH Bath Road RG7 5HT **BERKSHIRE**
☎ Reading (0734) 714411
PADWORTH COURT ★★★ **70%**
Access through main double swing doors from
Bath Road via ramp. Grab rails around bath only

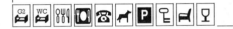

READING Caversham Bridge **BERKSHIRE**
Richfield Avenue RG1 8BD ☎ (0734) 391818
CAVERSHAM ★★★★ **60%**
Access through main double automatic doors
from Richfield Avenue via ramp

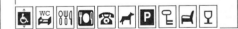

READING 387 Basingstoke Road **BERKSHIRE**
RG2 0JE
☎ (0734) 750618 Central Res (0800) 850950
FORTE TRAVELODGE ⌂
Access through main double doors from car park
via ramp

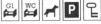

★★★★ hotel rating (see p.43)	⊠ Red highest award to Star hotel (see p.44)	% percentage rating (see p.44)	♣ country house hotel (see p.44)	⌂ travel lodge (see p.43)
GH guest house	T&C town & country homes (see p.42)	G1 ground floor bedrooms (A-annexe)	WC toilets *en suite*	access to reception
FH farmhouse	lift	guide dogs	dining room	access to lounge
INN inn	telephone/ intercom	P parking at entrance	room service	access to bar

* Details have not been confirmed for 1993. Please check when booking, including information about grab rails.

49

READING Oxford Road **BERKSHIRE**
RG1 7RH ☎ (0734) 586222
RAMADA ★★★★ 60%
Access through main doors from Oxford Road

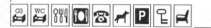

SLOUGH Ditton Road Langley **BERKSHIRE**
SL3 8PT ☎ (0753) 544244
HEATHROW/SLOUGH MARRIOTT ★★★★ 64%
Access through rear double swing doors from
Ditton Road via ramp

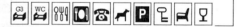

THATCHAM Bowling Green Road **BERKSHIRE**
RG13 3RP ☎ Newbury (0635) 871555
REGENCY PARK ★★★★ 63%
Access through main double doors from Bowling
Green Road

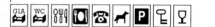

ASTON CLINTON* **BUCKINGHAMSHIRE**
HP22 5HP ☎ Aylesbury (0296) 630252
BELL INN ★★★ 78%
Access through main single door from London
Road via one step

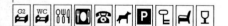

AYLESBURY **BUCKINGHAMSHIRE**
Aston Clinton Road HP22 5AA ☎ (0296) 393388
FORTE CREST ★★★★ 65%
Access through main double sliding doors off
Aston Clinton Road

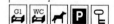

HIGH WYCOMBE **BUCKINGHAMSHIRE**
Handy Cross HP11 1TL ☎ (0494) 442100
FORTE POSTHOUSE ★★★ 65%
Access through main automatic doors

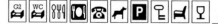

MILTON KEYNES **BUCKINGHAMSHIRE**
London Road Moulsoe MK16 0JA
☎ Newport Pagnell (0908) 613688
COACH HOUSE ★★★ 67%
Access through double side door via ramp

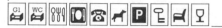

ALWALTON A1 **CAMBRIDGESHIRE**
Great North Road ☎ Peterborough (0733) 231109
Central Res (0800) 850950
FORTE TRAVELODGE ⌂
Access through main double doors from car park
via ramp

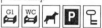

ALWALTON Lynchwood **CAMBRIDGESHIRE**
PE2 0GB ☎ Peterborough (0733) 371111
SWALLOW ★★★★ 64%
Access through main double sliding door

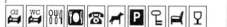

CAMBRIDGE Lakeview **CAMBRIDGESHIRE**
Bridge Road Impington CB4 4PH ☎ (0223) 237000
FORTE POSTHOUSE ★★★ 64%
Access through main automatic doors from Bridge
Road via two steps

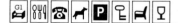

LOLWORTH Huntingdon **CAMBRIDGESHIRE**
Road CB3 8DR (on A604)
☎ Crafts Hill (0954) 781335 Central Res (0800) 850950
FORTE TRAVELODGE ⌂
Access through main double doors from car park
via ramp

PETERBOROUGH **CAMBRIDGESHIRE**
Thorpe Wood PE3 6SG ☎ (0733) 260000
PETERBOROUGH MOAT HOUSE ★★★ 68%
Access through main double swing doors from
Thorpe Wood via ramp

ST IVES Bridge Foot **CAMBRIDGESHIRE**
London Road PE17 4EP ☎ (0480) 66966
DOLPHIN ★★★ 62%
Access through main double swing doors from
London Road

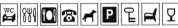

CHESTER* Eastgate Street **CHESHIRE**
CH1 1LT ☎ (0244) 324024
THE CHESTER GROSVENOR ★★★★ Red
Access through double swing doors from Eastgate
Street via ramp

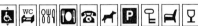

WISBECH **CAMBRIDGESHIRE**
West Drove North Walton Highway PE14 7DP
☎ (0945) 880162
STRATTON FARM FH
Access through main single door from West Drove
North via one step

CHESTER* Parkgate Road **CHESHIRE**
Mollington CH1 6NE ☎ (0244) 851666
CRABWELL MANOR ★★★ 78%
Access through main double swing doors from
Parkgate Road via ramp

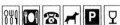

ADLINGTON A523 **CHESHIRE**
Adlington SK12 4NA
☎ (0625) 875292 Central Res (0800) 850950
FORTE TRAVELODGE ⌂
Access through main double doors from car park
via ramp

CHESTER Hoole Road CH2 3ND **CHESHIRE**
☎ (0244) 321165
DENE ★★ 62%
Access through main double swing doors from
Hoole Road via ramp. No grab rails in bathroom

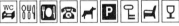

BRAMHALL Bramhall Lane South **CHESHIRE**
SK7 2EB ☎ 061-439 8116
BRAMHALL MOAT HOUSE ★★★ 68%
Access through main electric sliding door from
Bramhall Lane South

CHESTER Warrington Road **CHESHIRE**
CH2 3PD ☎ (0244) 350011
HOOLE HALL ★★★ 64%
Access through main double swing doors from
Warrington Road

BUCKLOW HILL* WA16 6RD **CHESHIRE**
☎ (0565) 830295
THE SWAN ★★★ 61%
Access through main single door from Chester
Road via one step

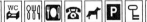

CHESTER Trinity Street CH1 2BD **CHESHIRE**
☎ (0244) 322330
MOAT HOUSE INTERNATIONAL ★★★★ 71%
Access through main double swing doors from car
park off Trinity Street via ramp

CHESTER Whitchurch Road **CHESHIRE**
Rowton CH3 6AD ☎ (0244) 335262
ROWTON HALL ★★★ **66%**
*Access through main single revolving doors from
Whitchurch Road*

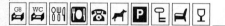

CREWE Sydney Road CW1 1LU **CHESHIRE**
☎ (0270) 583440
HUNTERS LODGE ★★★ **62%**
*Access through single door from Sydney Road. No
grab rails in bathroom*

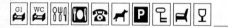

FRODSHAM Overton Hill **CHESHIRE**
WA6 6HH ☎ (0928) 35255
**FOREST HILL HOTEL
& LEISURE COMPLEX** ★★★ **64%**
*Access through main double swing doors from
Bellemonte Rd via one step. No grab rails in bathrm*

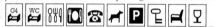

HOLMES CHAPEL Knutsford Road **CHESHIRE**
CW4 8EF ☎ (0477) 32041
OLD VICARAGE ★★★ **67%**
*Access through main double doors from
Knutsford Road*

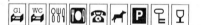

KNUTSFORD Manchester Road **CHESHIRE**
WA16 0SU ☎ (0565) 650333
COTTONS ★★★ **69%**
*Access through side double doors from
Manchester Road via one step*

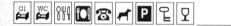

KNUTSFORD Chester Road **CHESHIRE**
Tabley WA16 0PP
☎ (0565) 652187 Central Res (0800) 850950
FORTE TRAVELODGE ⌂
*Access through main double doors from car park
via ramp*

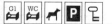

MACCLESFIELD Park Lane **CHESHIRE**
SK11 8AE ☎ (0625) 511428
PARK VILLA ★★ **65%**
*Access through rear single door from Woodlands
Road*

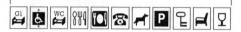

MOTTRAM ST ANDREW **CHESHIRE**
Wilmslow Road Prestbury SK10 4QT
☎ Prestbury (0625) 828135
MOTTRAM HALL ★★★★ **63%**
*Access through main double doors from
Wilmslow Road*

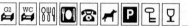

NANTWICH Worleston **CHESHIRE**
CW5 6DQ ☎ (0270) 610016
ROOKERY HALL ★★★ **80%** ♨
*Access through main single door via one step.
Grab rails around toilet only*

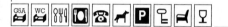

RUNCORN Lowlands Road **CHESHIRE**
WA7 5TP ☎ (0928) 581771
CAMPANILE ⌂
Access through main single door via ramp

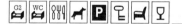

SANDBACH Congleton Road **CHESHIRE**
CW11 0ST ☎ Crewe (0270) 764141
CHIMNEY HOUSE ★★★ **65%**
Access through main double door

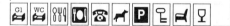

WARRINGTON **CHESHIRE**
Alexandra Road WA4 2EL ☎ (0925) 262898
ROCKFIELD ★★ **70%**
*Access through single door from Alexandra Road.
No grab rails in bathroom*

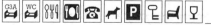

HARTLEPOOL* **CLEVELAND**
5/7 The Front Seaton Carew TS25 1BS
☎ (0429) 266244
THE MARINE ★★★ 55%
Access through side double doors from the car park via ramp

   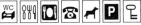 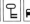

STOCKTON-ON-TEES **CLEVELAND**
636 Yarm Road TS16 0DH ☎ (0642) 786815
PARKMORE ★★★ 70%
Access through main double swing doors from Yarm Road via ramp. No grab rails in bathroom

FALMOUTH Western Terrace **CORNWALL**
TR11 4QJ ☎ (0326) 312734
GREEN LAWNS ★★★ 63%
Access through rear single door from Western Terrace via ramp. Grab rails around bath only

NEWQUAY* Porthway TR7 3LW **CORNWALL**
☎ (0637) 873274
PORTH VEOR MANOR HOUSE ★★ 59%
Access through main single door via one step

PORT ISAAC 4 New Road **CORNWALL**
PL29 3SB ☎ Bodmin (0208) 880300
CASTLE ROCK ★★ 64%
Access through rear single door from car park via one step. No grab rails in bathroom

REDRUTH* Scourrier TR16 5BP **CORNWALL**
☎ (0209) 820551
CROSSROADS ★★ 68%
Access through main/single door via ramp

ST AUSTELL 60 Alexandra Road **CORNWALL**
PL25 4QN ☎ (0726) 65707
SELWOOD HOUSE ★ 65%
Access through main single door from Alexandra Road via one step

SALTASH Callington Road **CORNWALL**
Carkeel PL12 6LF ☎ (0752) 848408
GRANADA LODGE ⌂
Access through main double doors from Callington Road via ramp

TREYARNON BAY PL28 8JW **CORNWALL**
☎ Padstow (0841) 520292
WATERBEACH ★★ 65%
Access through single door from car park via ramp

ALSTON* CA9 3JX **CUMBRIA**
☎ (0434) 381230
LOWBYER MANOR COUNTRY HOUSE ★★ 68%
Access through side and main single doors from Station Road via one step

AMBLESIDE Borrans Road **CUMBRIA**
LA22 0EN ☎ (05394) 33454
BORRANS PARK ★★ 69%
Access through double doors from car park

CONISTON Yewdale Road **CUMBRIA**
LA21 8DU ☎ (05394) 41335
BLACK BULL ★★ 63%
Access through main double doors from Yewdale Road

AMBLESIDE Rothay Bridge **CUMBRIA**
LA22 0EH ☎ (05394) 33605
ROTHAY MANOR ★★★ 73%
Access through main single doors via ramp

KESWICK Portinscale CA12 5RE **CUMBRIA**
☎ (07687) 72538
DERWENTWATER ★★★ 58%
Access through main single door. No grab rails in bathroom

APPLEBY-IN-WESTMORLAND **CUMBRIA**
Roman Road CA16 6JD ☎ (07683) 51571
**APPLEBY MANOR
COUNTRY HOUSE HOTEL ★★★ 70% ♨**
Access through side single door from Roman Road. Grab rails around bath only

NEWBY BRIDGE LA12 8AT **CUMBRIA**
☎ (05395) 31207
LAKESIDE ★★★ 70%
Access through main double doors from Hawkshead Road via ramp

CARLISLE 32 Scotland Road **CUMBRIA**
CA3 9DG ☎ (0228) 22887
CUMBRIA PARK ★★★ 66%
Access through single door from car park

PENRITH Redhills CA11 0DT **CUMBRIA**
☎ (0768) 66958 Central Res (0800) 850950
FORTE TRAVELODGE ⌂
Access through main double doors from car park via ramp

CARLISLE* London Road CA1 2PQ **CUMBRIA**
☎ (0228) 29255
SWALLOW HILLTOP ★★★ 59%
Access through side double doors from London Road via ramp

RAVENGLASS* CA18 1SD **CUMBRIA**
☎ (0229) 717222
PENNINGTON ARMS ★ 59%
Access through main single door from Main Street via ramp

CASTERTON LA6 2RX **CUMBRIA**
☎ Kirkby Lonsdale (05242) 71230
PHEASANT INN ★★ 69%
Access through single door from car park. Grab rails around toilets only

RAVENSTONEDALE* CA17 4NG **CUMBRIA**
☎ Newbiggin-on-Lune (05396) 23204
BLACK SWAN ★★ 70%
Access through side rear single door from car park via ramp

RAVENSTONEDALE Crossbank **CUMBRIA**
CA17 4LL ☎ Newbiggin-on-Lune (05396) 23242
THE FAT LAMB ★★ **65%**
*Access through rear single door. No grab rails in
bathroom*

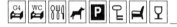

SHAP CA10 3QU **CUMBRIA**
☎ (0931) 716628
SHAP WELLS ★★ **66%**
Access through main double swing doors

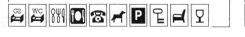

SOUTHWAITE MOTORWAY **CUMBRIA**
SERVICE AREA Bradfield Site CA4 0NT (on M6)
☎ (06974) 73131
GRANADA LODGE ⌂
Access through main double swing doors

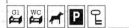

TEMPLE SOWERBY CA10 1RZ **CUMBRIA**
☎ Kirkby Thore (07683) 61578
TEMPLE SOWERBY HOUSE HOTEL ★★ **73%**
Access through side single door

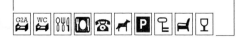

WATERMILLOCK CA11 0TH **CUMBRIA**
☎ Pooley Bridge (07684) 86038
WATERSIDE HOUSE GH
*Access through single door through main or rear
entrance*

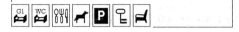

WETHERAL CA4 8ES **CUMBRIA**
☎ (0228) 561888
CROWN ★★★ **67%**
*Access through double doors from car park off
Station Road*

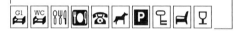

WINDERMERE Back Belsfield Road **CUMBRIA**
Bowness LA23 3HH ☎ (05394) 46226
BURN HOW GARDEN HOUSE ★★★ **67%**
*Access through main swing door from Back
Belsfield Road via ramp*

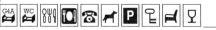

WINDERMERE Lake Road LA23 2JJ **CUMBRIA**
☎ (05394) 43624
WHITE LODGE GH
*Access through rear swing door from Lake Road
via one step*

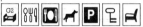

ALFRETON **DERBYSHIRE**
Old Swanwick Colliery Road (jnct A38/A61)
DE55 1HJ ☎ (0773) 520040
GRANADA LODGE ★★★ **58%**
*Access through main double doors from Old
Swanwick Colliery Road*

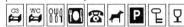

ASHBOURNE Derby Road **DERBYSHIRE**
DE6 1XH ☎ (0335) 46666
ASHBOURNE OAKS LODGE ★★★ **69%**
*Access through main double doors from Derby
Road*

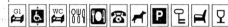

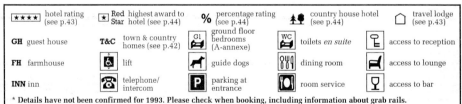

55

BAKEWELL Great Longstone **DERBYSHIRE**
DE45 1TF ☎ Great Longstone (0629) 640278
CROFT COUNTRY HOUSE HOTEL ★★ **73%** ♨
Access through main single door via two steps. No grab rails in bathroom

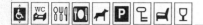

SOUTH NORMANTON **DERBYSHIRE**
Carter Lane East DE55 2EH ☎ Ripley (0773) 812000
SWALLOW ★★★★ **62%**
Access through main double doors from Carter Lane East

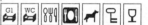

BUXTON 18 Broad Walk **DERBYSHIRE**
SK17 6JR ☎ (0298) 22638
HARTINGTON ★ **63%**
Access through main single door from Hartington Road

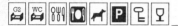

ASHBURTON TQ13 7NS **DEVON**
☎ Poundsgate (03643) 471
HOLNE CHASE ★★ **71%**
Access through main double doors

DERBY Pasture Hill **DERBYSHIRE**
Littleover DE23 7BA ☎ (0332) 514933
FORTE POSTHOUSE ★★★ **63%**
Access through main double swing doors via ramp. Guide dogs not allowed in the restaurant

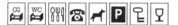

ASHBURTON* 68-70 East Street **DEVON**
TQ13 7AX ☎ (0364) 52206
TUGELA HOUSE ★★ **67%**
Access through main single door from East Street via ramp

LONG EATON* 20 Derby Road **DERBYSHIRE**
NG10 1LW ☎ (0602) 728481
EUROPA ★★ **60%**
Access through main single door from Derby Road via one step

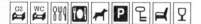

BARNSTAPLE Bickington Road **DEVON**
EX31 2HP ☎ (0271) 71784
CEDARS LODGE INN ⌂
Access through single swing door from car park

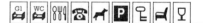

LONG EATON Bostock Lane **DERBYSHIRE**
NG10 5NL ☎ Nottingham (0602) 460000
SLEEP INN ★★ **67%**
Access through main double doors

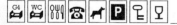

COLYTON* Dolphin Street EX13 6NA **DEVON**
☎ (0297) 552401
WHITE COTTAGE ★★ **65%**
Access through main single door from Dolphin Street

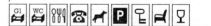

ROWSLEY DE4 2EF **DERBYSHIRE**
☎ Matlock (0629) 733949
EAST LODGE
COUNTRY HOUSE HOTEL ★★★ **64%**
Access through main single door from Matlock Road

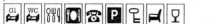

DAWLISH Dawlish Warren EX7 0NA **DEVON**
☎ (0626) 865155
LANGSTONE CLIFF ★★★ **60%**
Access through main double doors from Mount Pleasant

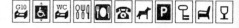

EXETER Southernhay East EX1 1QF	DEVON

EXETER Southernhay East EX1 1QF — DEVON
☎ (0392) 412812
FORTE CREST ★★★★ 67%
Access through main automatic sliding doors via ramp

[icons: G2 bed | WC toilets en suite | dining room | room service | telephone | guide dogs | P parking | access to reception | access to lounge | access to bar]

PLYMOUTH Marsh Mills — DEVON
Longbridge Road PL6 8LD ☎ (0752) 601087
CAMPANILE ⌂
Access through main single door from Longbridge Road

[icons: G2 bed | bed | dining room | room service | guide dogs | P parking | access to reception | access to lounge | access to bar]

EXETER Moor Lane Sandygate — DEVON
EX2 4AR ☎ (0392) 74044
GRANADA ★★★ 63%
Access through double doors from car park

[icons: G2 bed | WC toilets en suite | dining room | room service | telephone | guide dogs | P parking | access to reception | access to lounge | access to bar]

PLYMOUTH Armada Way PL1 1AR — DEVON
☎ (0752) 224161
COPTHORNE ★★★★ 65%
Access through side double swing doors from Armada Way via ramp

[icons: lift | WC toilets en suite | dining room | room service | telephone | guide dogs | P parking | access to reception | access to lounge | access to bar]

HAYTOR TQ13 9XX — DEVON
☎ (0364) 661217
BEL ALP HOUSE ★★★ 77%
Access through main single door from car park via two steps. No grab rails in bathroom

[icons: G2 bed | lift | WC toilets en suite | dining room | room service | telephone | guide dogs | P parking | access to reception | access to lounge | access to bar]

PLYMOUTH* Marsh Mills Roundabout — DEVON
270 Plymouth Road PL6 8NH ☎ (0752) 221422
NOVOTEL PLYMOUTH ★★★ 58%
Access through main automatic sliding doors via ramp

[icons: G2 bed | bed | dining room | room service | telephone | guide dogs | P parking | access to reception | access to lounge | access to bar]

HORRABRIDGE PL20 7RN — DEVON
☎ Yelverton (0822) 853501
OVERCOMBE ★★ 67%
Access through rear single door from Station Road via ramp

[icons: G1 bed | WC toilets en suite | dining room | room service | guide dogs | P parking | access to reception | access to lounge | access to bar]

PLYMOUTH* Armada Way PL1 2HJ — DEVON
☎ (0752) 662866
PLYMOUTH MOAT HOUSE ★★★★ 60%
Access through main double doors from Armada Way via ramp

[icons: G2 bed | lift | WC toilets en suite | dining room | room service | telephone | guide dogs | P parking | access to reception | access to lounge | access to bar]

OKEHAMPTON Sourton Cross — DEVON
EX20 4LY ☎ (0837) 52124 Central Res (0800) 850950
FORTE TRAVELODGE ⌂
Access through main double doors from car park via ramp

[icons: G1 bed | WC toilets en suite | guide dogs | P parking | access to reception]

ROUSDON* DT7 3XW — DEVON
☎ Lyme Regis (0297) 442972
ORCHARD COUNTRY ★★ 64%
Access through rear double doors from Comlapyne Road via one step

[icons: G2 bed | WC toilets en suite | dining room | guide dogs | P parking | access to reception | access to lounge | access to bar]

SAMPFORD PEVERELL Sampford   **DEVON**
Peverell Service Area EX16 7HD (SE jct 27 M5)
☎ Tiverton (0884) 821087 Central Res (0800) 850950
FORTE TRAVELODGE ⌂
*Access through main double doors from car park
via ramp*

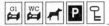

BOURNEMOUTH Richmond Hill   **DORSET**
BH2 6EN ☎ (0202) 551521
NORFOLK ROYALE ★★★★ **69%**
*Access through main double swing doors from
Richmond Hill via ramp.*
No grab rails in bathrooms

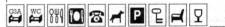

TIVERTON Blundells Road EX16 4DB   **DEVON**
☎ (0884) 256120
TIVERTON ★★★ **61%**
*Access through main double swing doors from
Blundells Road via ramp*

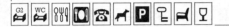

BRIDPORT West Bay DT6 4EL   **DORSET**
☎ (0308) 23626
HADDON HOUSE ★★★ **61%**
Access through main double doors

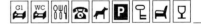

TORQUAY Herbert Road Chelston   **DEVON**
TQ2 6RW ☎ (0803) 605446
FAIRMOUNT HOUSE ★ **70%**
*Access through side single door from Herbert
Road via ramp. Grab rails around toilets only*

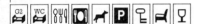

EVERSHOT* DT2 0JR   **DORSET**
☎ (0935) 83424
SUMMER LODGE ★★★ Red ♨
Access through main single door via ramp

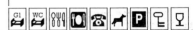

BLANDFORD FORUM Church Road   **DORSET**
DT11 8UB ☎ (0258) 456756
FAIRFIELD HOUSE GH
*Access through main double doors from Church
Road via ramp*

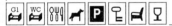

HORTON BH21 7HL   **DORSET**
☎ Witchampton (0258) 840407
NORTHILL HOUSE GH
Access through main single door

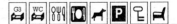

BOURNEMOUTH   **DORSET**
12-14 Knyveton Road BH1 3QP ☎ (0202) 293071
ELSTEAD ★★★ **65%**
*Access through main double doors from Knyveton
Road*

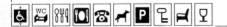

ST LEONARDS BH24 2NP   **DORSET**
☎ (0425) 471220
ST LEONARDS ★★★ **67%**
*Access through main double doors from
Ringwood Road*

BOURNEMOUTH   **DORSET**
16 Boscombe Spa Road BH5 1BB ☎ (0202) 302442
HOTEL COURTLANDS ★★★ **65%**
*Access through main double doors from
Boscombe Spa Road via ramp.*
Grab rails around baths only

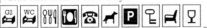

STURMINSTER NEWTON   **DORSET**
Lydlinch DT10 2JB
☎ Hazelbury Bryan (0258) 817348
HOLEBROOK FARM FH
Access through main single door via ramp

SWANAGE Burlington Road   **DORSET**
BH19 1LT ☎ (0929) 425211
PINES ★★★ **62%**
Access through main double doors from
Burlington Road via ramp

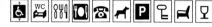

WAREHAM East Stoke BH20 6AL   **DORSET**
☎ Bindon Abbey (0929) 462563
KEMPS COUNTRY HOUSE ★★ **69%**
Access through double doors

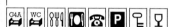

DURHAM Old Elvet DH1 3JN   **CO DURHAM**
☎ 091-386 6821
SWALLOW ★★★★ **68%**
Access through main doors from Old Elvet

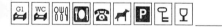

THORNLEY Dunelm Road   **CO DURHAM**
DH6 3HT ☎ (0429) 821248
CROSSWAYS ★★ **64%**
Access through main double doors from Dunelm
Road

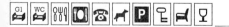

COODEN BEACH TN39 4TT   **EAST SUSSEX**
☎ (04243) 2281
COODEN RESORT ★★★ **64%**
Access through rear double swing doors from
Herbrand Walk via ramp

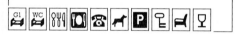

EASTBOURNE   **EAST SUSSEX**
King Edwards Parade BN21 4EQ ☎ (0323) 412345
GRAND ★★★★★ **65%**
Access through main double and revolving doors
from King Edward's Parade via ramp. No grab
rails in bathroom

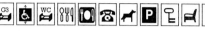

HAILSHAM A22   **EAST SUSSEX**
Hellingly BN27 4DT
☎ (0323) 844556 Central Res (0800) 850950
FORTE TRAVELODGE ⌂
Access through main double doors from car park
via ramp

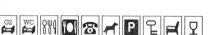

PEVENSEY* Castle Road   **EAST SUSSEX**
BN24 5LG ☎ Eastbourne (0323) 763150
PRIORY COURT ★★ **58%**
Access through rear single door from car park via
one step

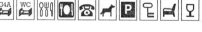

UCKFIELD Little Horsted   **EAST SUSSEX**
TN22 5TS ☎ Isfield (0825) 750581
HORSTED PLACE ★★★ Red ⚘
Access through side single door via ramp. Grab
rails in bathroom around baths but not toilets

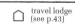

BASILDON Pipps Hill   **ESSEX**
Southend Arterial Road SS14 3AE
☎ (0268) 530810
CAMPANILE ⌂
Access through main single swing doors from
Miles Gray Road

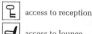

★★★★	hotel rating (see p.43)	⊡ Red Star	highest award to hotel (see p.44)	%	percentage rating (see p.44)	⚘	country house hotel (see p.44)	⌂	travel lodge (see p.43)
GH	guest house	**T&C**	town & country homes (see p.42)	G1 ⊨	ground floor bedrooms (A-annexe)	WC ⊨	toilets *en suite*	⊑	access to reception
FH	farmhouse	ⓐ	lift	⟂	guide dogs	⦀	dining room	⊨	access to lounge
INN	inn	☎	telephone/ intercom	**P**	parking at entrance	⦿	room service	ⵝ	access to bar

* Details have not been confirmed for 1993. Please check when booking, including information about grab rails.

BASILDON Felmores East Mayne **ESSEX**
SS13 1BW ☎ (0268) 522227
WATERMILL TRAVEL INN ⌂
Access through main single door from Burnt Mills Road

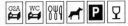

BRENTWOOD London Road **ESSEX**
CM14 4NR ☎ (0277) 225252
BRENTWOOD MOAT HOUSE ★★★★ 65%
Access through main double doors from London Road

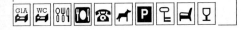

COLCHESTER London Road **ESSEX**
CO6 1DU ☎ (0206) 210001
MARKS TEY ★★★ 67%
Access through main double doors from London Road via ramp

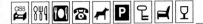

EAST HORNDON CM13 3LL **ESSEX**
☎ Brentwood (0277) 810819 Central Res (0800) 850950
FORTE TRAVELODGE ⌂
Access through main double doors from car park via ramp

INGATESTONE* Roman Road **ESSEX**
CM4 9AB ☎ (0277) 355355
HEYBRIDGE MOAT HOUSE ★★★ 63%
Access through side swing door from Roman Road via one step

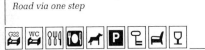

WALTHAM ABBEY Old Shire Lane **ESSEX**
EN9 3LX ☎ Lea Valley (0992) 717170
SWALLOW ★★★★ 63%
Access through main swing doors

WEST THURROCK RM16 3BG **ESSEX**
☎ (0708) 891111
GRANADA LODGE ⌂
Access through main automatic door via ramp

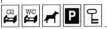

BIRDLIP GL4 8JH **GLOUCESTERSHIRE**
☎ Gloucester (0452) 862506
ROYAL GEORGE ★★★ 63%
Access through main double swing door via one step. No grab rails in bathroom

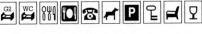

BOURTON-ON-THE- **GLOUCESTERSHIRE**
WATER Victoria Street
GL54 2BU ☎ Cotswold (0451) 820286
CHESTER HOUSE ★★ 64%
Access through single door from car park off Victoria Road via ramp

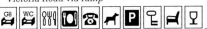

CHELTENHAM **GLOUCESTERSHIRE**
Shurdington GL51 5UG ☎ (0242) 862352
GREENWAY ★★★ Red ♨
Access through main double doors via ramp. No grab rails in bathroom

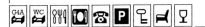

CHELTENHAM **GLOUCESTERSHIRE**
The Burgage Prestbury GL52 3DN
☎ (0242) 529533
PRESTBURY HOUSE ★★★ 62%
Access through main single door from The Burgage via ramp

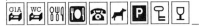

CHIPPING CAMPDEN **GLOUCESTERSHIRE**
High Street GL55 6AT ☎ Evesham (0386) 840317
NOEL ARMS ★★ 69%
Access through side double doors through conservatory from High Street

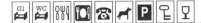

CIRENCESTER — **GLOUCESTERSHIRE**
Ampney Crucis GL7 5RS ☎ (0285) 851806
CROWN OF CRUCIS ★★★ **63%**
Access through double doors from the car park via ramp

  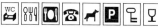

CLEARWELL GL16 8JT — **GLOUCESTERSHIRE**
☎ Dean (0594) 833666
WYNDHAM ARMS ★★★ **64%**
Access through side double doors. No grab rails in bathroom

  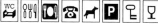

FAIRFORD — **GLOUCESTERSHIRE**
London Street GL7 4AH
☎ Cirencester (0285) 712349
HYPERION HOUSE ★★★ **58**
Access through single doors from car park off London Street. No grab rails in bathroom

TETBURY — **GLOUCESTERSHIRE**
London Road GL8 8JJ ☎ (0666) 502251
PRIORY INN ★★★ **62%**
Access through main double doors from car park off London Road via ramp. No grab rails in bathroom

 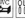 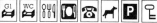

BOLTON — **GREATER MANCHESTER**
1 Higher Bridge Street BL1 2EW ☎ (0204) 383338
MOAT HOUSE ★★★ **70%**
Access through main double automatic doors from Higher Bridge Street via ramp

  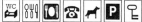

BOLTON — **GREATER MANCHESTER**
Bradshawgate BL1 1DP ☎ (0204) 27261
PACK HORSE ★★★ **60%**
Access through main double doors from Nelson Square via one step. No grab rails in bathroom

BURY — **GREATER MANCHESTER**
Walshaw Road BL8 1PU ☎ 061-764 3888
BOLHOLT ★★ **64%**
Access through main double swing doors from Walshaw Road via ramp

MANCHESTER — **GREATER MANCHESTER**
Peter Street M60 2DS ☎ 061-236 3333
HOLIDAY INN CROWNE PLAZA ★★★★ **67%**
Access through main door from Peter Street

STANDISH — **GREATER MANCHESTER**
Almond Brook Road WN6 0SR ☎ (0257) 425588
ALMOND BROOK MOAT HOUSE ★★★ **64%**
Access through main automatic double doors from Almond Brook Road

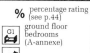 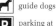

AMPFIELD SO51 9ZF — **HAMPSHIRE**
☎ Southampton (0703) 266611
POTTERS HERON ★★★ **66%**
Access through main single and double doors via ramp

ANDOVER Micheldever Road	**HAMPSHIRE**
☎ (0264) 357344
ASHLEY COURT ★★★ **61%**
Access through main double swing doors from Micheldever Road via ramp

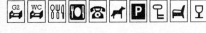

EASTLEIGH Twyford Road	**HAMPSHIRE**
☎ (0703) 616813 Central Res (0800) 850950
FORTE TRAVELODGE ⌂
Access through main double doors from car park via ramp

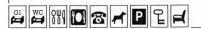

BARTON STACEY	**HAMPSHIRE**
SO21 3NP (on A303)
☎ Andover (0264) 72260 Central Res (0800) 850950
FORTE TRAVELODGE ⌂
Access through main double doors from car park via ramp

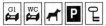

FAREHAM 22 The Avenue	**HAMPSHIRE**
PO14 1NS ☎ (0329) 232175
AVENUE HOUSE GH
Access through main single door from The Avenue via ramp. Only breakfast served

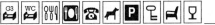

BASINGSTOKE Nately Scures	**HAMPSHIRE**
Hook RG27 JS ☎ (0256) 764161
BASINGSTOKE COUNTRY HOTEL ★★★ **67%**
Access through main automatic sliding doors from London Road

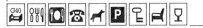

FAREHAM Cartwright Drive	**HAMPSHIRE**
PO15 5RJ ☎ (0329) 844644
FORTE POSTHOUSE ★★★ **68%**
Access through main double swing doors from Cartwright Drive via ramp

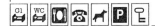

BASINGSTOKE* Grove Road	**HAMPSHIRE**
RG21 3EE
FORTE POSTHOUSE ★★★ **31%**
Access through main swing doors from Grove Road via one step

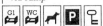

FAREHAM East Street	**HAMPSHIRE**
PO16 0BP ☎ (0329) 822640
RED LION ★★ **68%**
Access through main double doors from East Street. Grab rails around bath only

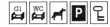

BASINGSTOKE Stag and Hounds	**HAMPSHIRE**
Winchester Road RG22 6HN
☎ (0256) 843566 Central Res (0800) 850950
FORTE TRAVELODGE ⌂
Access through main double doors from car park via ramp

FOUR MARKS	**HAMPSHIRE**
156 Winchester Road GU34 5HZ (on A31)
☎ Alton (0420) 62659 Central Res (0800) 850950
FORTE TRAVELODGE ⌂
Access through main double doors from car park via ramp

BROOK SO43 7HE	**HAMPSHIRE**
☎ Southampton (0703) 812214
BELL INN ★★★ **69%**
Access through main double door via ramp

HOOK Station Road RG27 9HS	**HAMPSHIRE**
☎ (0256) 762541
RAVEN ★★ **67%**
Access through main double doors from Station Road via ramp

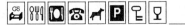

LEE-ON-THE-SOLENT **HAMPSHIRE**
39 Marine Parade East PO13 9BW ☎ (0705) 550258
BELLE VUE HOTEL ★★★ 64%
Access through double swing doors from east car
park off Marine Parade East.
No grab rails in bathrooms

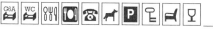

SUTTON SCOTNEY SO21 3JY **HAMPSHIRE**
(A34 Northbound) ☎ Winchester (0962) 761016
Central Res (0800) 850950
FORTE TRAVELODGE ⌂
Access through main double doors from car park
via ramp

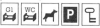

MIDDLE WALLOP SO20 8EG **HAMPSHIRE**
☎ Andover (0264) 781565
FIFEHEAD MANOR ★★ 68%
Access through rear swing doors

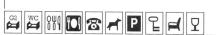

SUTTON SCOTNEY SO21 3JY **HAMPSHIRE**
(A34 Southbound) ☎ Winchester (0962) 760779
Central Res (0800) 850950
FORTE TRAVELODGE ⌂
Access through main double doors from car park
via ramp

NORTH WALTHAM RG25 2BB **HAMPSHIRE**
☎ Dummer (0256) 398282
WHEATSHEAF ★★ 65%
Access through main double doors from car park

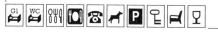

WINCHESTER Sparsholt **HAMPSHIRE**
SO21 2LT (3m NW off A272) ☎ (0962) 863588
LAINSTON HOUSE ★★★★ 71%
Access through main double doors. No grab rails
in bathroom

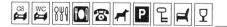

PORTSMOUTH Pembroke Road **HAMPSHIRE**
PO1 2TA ☎ (0705) 827651
FORTE POSTHOUSE ★★★ 68%
Access through automatic doors via ramp.
Grab rails around bath only

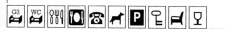

WINCHESTER 44 St Cross Street **HAMPSHIRE**
SO23 9PS ☎ (0962) 854901
MARLAND GH
Access through rear single door from car park off
Edgar Road

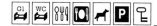

PORTSMOUTH North Harbour **HAMPSHIRE**
PO6 4SH ☎ (0705) 383151
PORTSMOUTH MARRIOTT ★★★ 68%
Access through main double electric doors from
Southampton Road via ramp

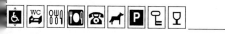

WINCHESTER Worthy Lane **HAMPSHIRE**
SO23 7AB ☎ (0962) 868102
WINCHESTER MOAT HOUSE ★★★ 68%
Access through main double swing doors from
Worthy Lane via ramp

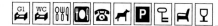

★★★★	hotel rating (see p.43)	⭐ Red Star	highest award to hotel (see p.44)	%	percentage rating (see p.44)	♣	country house hotel (see p.44)	⌂	travel lodge (see p.43)
GH	guest house	T&C	town & country homes (see p.42)	G1	ground floor bedrooms (A-annexe)	WC	toilets *en suite*		access to reception
FH	farmhouse		lift		guide dogs		dining room		access to lounge
INN	inn		telephone/ intercom	P	parking at entrance		room service		access to bar

* Details have not been confirmed for 1993. Please check when booking, including information about grab rails.

BROMSGROVE | **HEREFORD & WORCESTER**
Kidderminster Road B61 9AB ☎ (0527) 576600
PINE LODGE ★★★ **71%**
Access through main double automatic doors
from Kidderminster Road

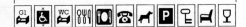

REDDITCH | **HEREFORD & WORCESTER**
Far Moor Lane Winyates Green B98 0SD
☎ (0527) 510710
CAMPANILE ⌂
Access through single door from car park off Far
Moor Lane

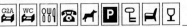

BROMSGROVE | **HEREFORD & WORCESTER**
Birmingham Road B61 0JB ☎ 021-447 7888
STAKIS BIRMINGHAM-BROMSGROVE
COUNTY COURT ★★★★ **65%**
Access through front main double doors

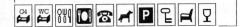

ROSS-ON-WYE | **HEREFORD & WORCESTER**
(4m N on A49 Hereford Road) HR9 6LL
☎ Harewood End (098987) 211
PENGETHLEY MANOR ★★★ **68%**
Access through main single door

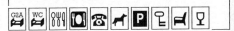

DROITWICH | **HEREFORD & WORCESTER**
Rashwood Hill WR9 8DA (on A38)
☎ Wychbold (052786) 545 Central Res (0800) 850950
FORTE TRAVELODGE ⌂
Access through main double doors from car park
via ramp

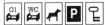

BALDOCK | **HERTFORDSHIRE**
Great North Road SG7 5EX (A1) ☎ Hinxworth
(0462) 835329 Central Res (0800) 850950
FORTE TRAVELODGE ⌂
Access through main double doors from car park
via ramp

HEREFORD | **HEREFORD & WORCESTER**
Belmont Road HR2 7BP ☎ (0432) 354301
HEREFORD MOAT HOUSE ★★★ **67%**
Access through main automatic sliding doors

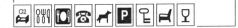

BOREHAMWOOD | **HERTFORDSHIRE**
Barnet Bypass WD6 5PU ☎ 081-953 1622
ELSTREE MOAT HOUSE ★★★★ **67%**
Access through main double automatic doors
from Barnet Bypass

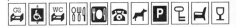

KIDDERMINSTER | **HEREFORD & WORCESTER**
Heath Lane Shenstone DY10 4BS ☎ (0562) 777535
GRANARY ★★★ **61%**
Access through main doors via ramp

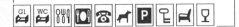

HATFIELD | **HERTFORDSHIRE**
Roehyde Way AL10 9AF ☎ (0707) 275701
HAZEL GROVE ★★★ **61%**
Access through main swing doors from Roehyde
Way via ramp

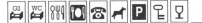

KIDDERMINSTER* | **HEREFORD & WORCESTER**
Stone DY10 4PJ ☎ (0562) 777555
STONE MANOR ★★★★ **55%**
Access through main double doors via one step

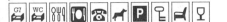

BEVERLEY* Tickton | **HUMBERSIDE**
HU17 9SH (3m NE on A1035)
☎ Hornsea (0964) 543666
TICKTON GRANGE ★★★ **63%**
Access through main double doors via one step

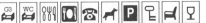

HULL Beverley Road   **HUMBERSIDE**
Freetown Way HU2 9AN ☎ (0482) 25530
CAMPANILE ⌂
Access through main single door via one step.
Grab rails around toilet only

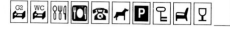

HULL Castle Street HU1 2BX   **HUMBERSIDE**
☎ (0482) 225221
FORTE CREST ★★★★ **61%**
Access through main double doors from Castle
Street

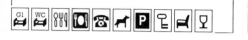

WILLERBY Mainstreet   **HUMBERSIDE**
HU10 6EA ☎ Hull (0482) 656488
GRANGE PARK ★★★ **71%**
Access through main double swing doors

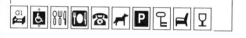

ASHFORD Simone Weil Avenue   **KENT**
TN24 8UX ☎ (0233) 611444
ASHFORD INTERNATIONAL HOTEL ★★★★ **67%**
Access through main automatic swing doors from
Simone Weil Avenue via ramp.
Grab rails around toilet only

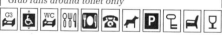

ASHFORD Eastwell Park   **KENT**
Boughton Lees TN25 4HR ☎ (0233) 635751
EASTWELL MANOR ★★★★ Red ▲♣
Access through main double doors from
Faversham Road via one step.
No grab rails in bathroom

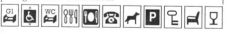

ASHFORD Canterbury Road   **KENT**
TN24 8QQ ☎ (0233) 625790
FORTE POSTHOUSE ★★★ **62%**
Access through main double swing doors from car
park off Canterbury Road

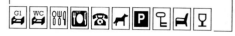

BRANDS HATCH DA3 8PE   **KENT**
☎ West Kingsdown (0474) 854900
BRANDS HATCH THISTLE ★★★★ **60%**
Access through main double swing doors via
ramp

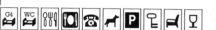

DOVER Singledge Lane   **KENT**
Whitfield CT16 3LF ☎ (0304) 821222
FORTE POSTHOUSE ★★★ **62%**
Access through main door from Singledge Avenue

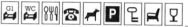

FARTHING CORNER MOTORWAY   **KENT**
SERVICE AREA M2 Motorway (between jncts 4 &
5) Hartlip ☎ Medway (0634) 377337
PAVILION LODGE ⌂
Access through main double doors via ramp

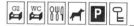

GRAVESEND Hever Court Road   **KENT**
DA12 5UQ ☎ (0474) 353100
SINGLEWELL MANOR HOTEL ★★★ **72%**
Access through main double doors from Hever
Court Road via ramp

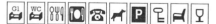

★★★★ hotel rating (see p.43)	★ Red highest award to Star hotel (see p.44)	% percentage rating (see p.44)
	▲♣ country house hotel (see p.44)	⌂ travel lodge (see p.43)
GH guest house	**T&C** town & country homes (see p.42)	G1 ground floor bedrooms (A-annexe)
	WC toilets *en suite*	⌷ access to reception
FH farmhouse	⚹ lift	guide dogs
	♨♨♨ dining room	access to lounge
INN inn	☎ telephone/ intercom	**P** parking at entrance
	room service	⍾ access to bar

* Details have not been confirmed for 1993. Please check when booking, including information about grab rails.

MAIDSTONE Bearsted Road Weavering **KENT**
ME14 5AA ☎ (0622) 34322 due to change to 734322
STAKIS MAIDSTONE
COUNTRY CLUB ★★★★ **65%**
Access through main double doors from Bearsted
Road via ramp

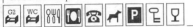

MAIDSTONE* Ashford Road **KENT**
Bearsted ME14 4NQ
☎ (0622) 34334 due to change to 734334
TUDOR PARK ★★★ **70%**
Access through main double doors from Ashford
Road via ramp

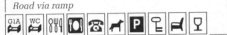

ROCHESTER Bridgewood Roundabout **KENT**
Maidstone Road ME5 9AX
☎ Medway (0634) 201333
BRIDGEWOOD MANOR ★★★★ **67%**
Access through main double doors via ramp

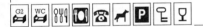

ROCHESTER Maidstone Road ME5 9SF **KENT**
☎ Medway (0634) 687111
FORTE POSTHOUSE ★★★ **68%**
Access through side double doors from Maidstone
Road via ramp

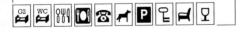

SHIPBOURNE Stumble Hill TN11 9PE **KENT**
☎ Plaxtol (0732) 810360
THE CHASER INN INN
Access through side single door from courtyard
via one step

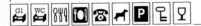

TONBRIDGE Pembury Road TN11 0NA **KENT**
☎ (0732) 773111
CHIMNEYS MOTOR INN ⌂
Access through main double door from Pembury
Road

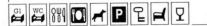

TUNBRIDGE WELLS (Royal)* **KENT**
Mount Ephraim TN4 8XJ ☎ (0892) 520331
SPA ★★★ **76%**
Access through main double doors from Mount
Ephraim via ramp

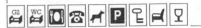

WATERINGBURY Tonbridge Road **KENT**
ME18 5NS ☎ Maidstone (0622) 812632
WATERINGBURY ★★★ **67%**
Access through main double doors

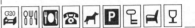

WROTHAM London Road Wrotham **KENT**
Heath TN15 7RS ☎ Borough Green (0732) 883311
FORTE POSTHOUSE
MAIDSTONE/SEVENOAKS ★★★ **65%**
Access through main double swing doors from
London Road via ramp

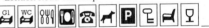

BURNLEY Calvalry Barracks **LANCASHIRE**
BB11 4AS ☎ (0282) 416039
Central Res (0800) 850950
FORTE TRAVELODGE ⌂
Access through main double doors from car park
via ramp

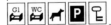

CHORLEY Preston Road **LANCASHIRE**
PR6 7AX ☎ (0257) 269966
HARTWOOD HALL ★★ **66%**
Access through single and double doors from
Preston Road. No grab rails in bathroom

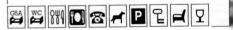

CLAYTON-LE-WOODS PR6 7ED **LANCASHIRE**
(1m S of M6 jnct 29 on A6)
☎ Preston (0722) 38551
PINES ★★★ **67%**
Access through single door from Preston Road. No
grab rails in bathroom

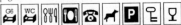

FORTON MOTORWAY SERVICE **LANCASHIRE**
AREA White Carr Lane Bay Horse LA2 9DU
☎ (0524) 792227
PAVILION LODGE ⌂
Access through main double doors via ramp

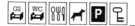

LYTHAM ST ANNES **LANCASHIRE**
South Promenade FY8 1NP
☎ (0253) 720061
CHADWICK ★★★ 68%
*Access through main single door from South
Promenade via ramp*

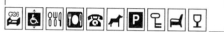

LANCASTER Waterside Park **LANCASHIRE**
Caton Road LA1 4RA ☎ (0524) 65999
FORTE POSTHOUSE ★★★ 63%
*Access through main automatic double doors
from Caton Road via ramp*

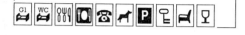

PRESTON Reedfield Place **LANCASHIRE**
PR5 6AB ☎ (0772) 313331
NOVOTEL ★★★ 57%
Access through main double doors

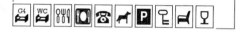

LANCASTER Green Lane **LANCASHIRE**
Ellel LA1 4GJ ☎ (0524) 844822
LANCASTER HOUSE ★★★ 73%
*Access through main double doors from Green
Lane*

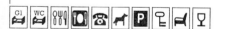

PRESTON Preston New Road **LANCASHIRE**
PR5 0UL ☎ (0772) 877351
SWALLOW TRAFALGAR ★★★ 62%
*Access through main double swing doors from
Preston New Road*

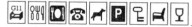

LANGHO Whalley Road **LANCASHIRE**
BB6 8AB ☎ Blackburn (0254) 240662
MYTTON FOLD FARM ★★★ 65%
*Access through main single door from Whalley
Road*

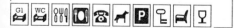

WRIGHTINGTON Moss Lane **LANCASHIRE**
WN6 9PB ☎ Standish (0257) 425803
**WRIGHTINGTON HOTEL
& RESTAURANT** ★★★ 65%
*Access through main double doors from Moss
Lane via one step*

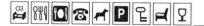

LEYLAND* Leyland Way **LANCASHIRE**
PR5 2JX ☎ Preston (0772) 422922
LEYLAND RESORT ★★★ 56%
Access through main double doors via one step

CASTLE DONINGTON **LEICESTERSHIRE**
East Midlands Airport DE7 2SH
☎ Derby (0332) 850700
DONINGTON THISTLE ★★★ 67%
Access through main double doors

★★★★	hotel rating (see p.43)	⋆ Red Star	highest award to hotel (see p.44)	%	percentage rating (see p.44)	♠♣	country house hotel (see p.44)	⌂	travel lodge (see p.43)
GH	guest house	**T&C**	town & country homes (see p.42)	G1	ground floor bedrooms (A-annexe)	WC	toilets *en suite*	⎾	access to reception
FH	farmhouse		lift		guide dogs		dining room		access to lounge
INN	inn		telephone/ intercom	**P**	parking at entrance		room service	♡	access to bar

* Details have not been confirmed for 1993. Please check when booking, including information about grab rails.

LEICESTER Wigston Road **LEICESTERSHIRE**
Oadby LE2 5QE ☎ (0533) 719441
LEICESTERSHIRE MOAT HOUSE ★★★ **65%**
Access through main triple swing doors from
Wigston Road

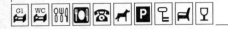

LEICESTER Hinckley Road **LEICESTERSHIRE**
Leicester Forest East LE3 3PG ☎ (0533) 387878
RED COW ★★ **69%**
Access through main double swing doors from
Hinckley Road via ramp

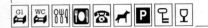

LEICESTER **LEICESTERSHIRE**
299 Leicester Road LE18 1JW ☎ (0533) 886161
STAGE ★★★ **63%**
Access through main double swing doors from car
park off Leicester Road via ramp

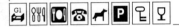

LEICESTER Braunstone **LEICESTERSHIRE**
LE3 2WQ ☎ (0533) 630066
STAKIS COUNTRY COURT ★★★★ **66%**
Access through main double doors

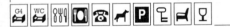

LUTTERWORTH* **LEICESTERSHIRE**
High Street LE17 4AD ☎ (0455) 553537
DENBIGH ARMS ★★★ **69%**
Access through main double doors via two steps

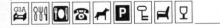

MARKFIELD Markfield Lane **LEICESTERSHIRE**
LE6 0PS ☎ (0530) 245454
FIELD HEAD ★★★ **71%**
Access through main double end swing doors via
ramp

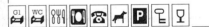

MARKFIELD **LEICESTERSHIRE**
Little Shaw Lane LE6 0PP
☎ Leicester (0530) 244237
GRANADA LODGE ⌂
Access through main double doors

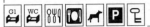

MELTON MOWBRAY **LEICESTERSHIRE**
Stapleford LE14 2EF ☎ Wymondham (057284) 522
STAPLEFORD PARK ★★★ Red ♨
Access through main single door from Stapleford
Road via ramp. Grab rails around toilet only

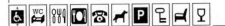

MELTON MOWBRAY **LEICESTERSHIRE**
Asfordby Road LE13 0HP ☎ (0664) 63563
SYSONBY KNOLL ★★ **62%**
Access through main double doors from Asfordby
Road

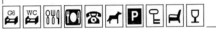

MORCOTT Uppingham **LEICESTERSHIRE**
LE15 8SA ☎ (0572) 87719 Central Res (0800)
850950
FORTE TRAVELODGE ⌂
Access through main double doors from car park
via ramp

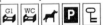

NORMANTON* LE15 8RP **LEICESTERSHIRE**
☎ Stamford (0780) 720315
NORMANTON PARK ★★★ **72%**
Access through main single door from car park
via ramp

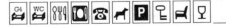

OAKHAM The Avenue **LEICESTERSHIRE**
Exton LE15 8AH ☎ (0572) 724678
BARNSDALE LODGE ★★★ **70%**
Access through main double doors from The
Avenue via ramp. Grab rails around bath only

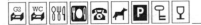

THRUSSINGTON **LEICESTERSHIRE**
Green Acres Filling Station LE7 8TE
☎ Rearsby (0664) 424525 Central Res (0800) 850950
FORTE TRAVELODGE ⌂
*Access through main double doors from car park
via ramp*

BRANSTON LN4 1HU **LINCOLNSHIRE**
☎ Lincoln (0522) 791366
MOOR LODGE ★★★ 54%
*Access through side single door from car park. No
grab rails in bathroom*

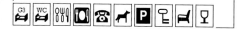

COLSTERWORTH NG33 5JJ **LINCOLNSHIRE**
(at junc A1/A151) ☎ Grantham (0476) 861181
Central Res (0800) 850950
FORTE TRAVELODGE ⌂
Access through main double doors from car park

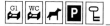

COLSTERWORTH (A1) **LINCOLNSHIRE**
NG33 5JR ☎ Grantham (0476) 860686
GRANADA LODGE ⌂
Access through main double doors

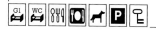

GRANTHAM **LINCOLNSHIRE**
Grantham Service Area NG32 2AB
☎ (0476) 77500 Central Res (0800) 850950
FORTE TRAVELODGE ⌂
*Access through main double doors from car park
via ramp*

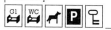

GRANTHAM North Parade **LINCOLNSHIRE**
NG31 8AU ☎ (0476) 590800
KINGS ★★ 66%
*Access through main double swing doors from
North Parade*

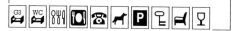

STAMFORD St Martins **LINCOLNSHIRE**
PE9 2LP ☎ (0780) 63359
GARDEN HOUSE ★★★ 69%
*Access through rear double doors from car park
via ramp. No grab rails in bathroom*

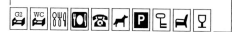

STAMFORD 37-38 High Street **LINCOLNSHIRE**
St Martins PE9 2LJ ☎ (0780) 481184
LADY ANNE'S ★★ 60%
*Access through double doors from car park. Grab
rails around bath only*

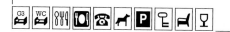

LONG SUTTON (A17) **LINCOLNSHIRE**
PE12 9AG ☎ (0406) 362230
Central Res (0800) 850950
FORTE TRAVELODGE ⌂
*Access through main double doors from car park
via ramp*

SLEAFORD A17/A15 **LINCOLNSHIRE**
Holdingham ☎ (0529) 414752
Central Res (0800) 850950
FORTE TRAVELODGE ⌂
*Access through main double doors from car park
via ramp*

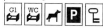

★★★★ hotel rating (see p.43)	★ Red highest award to Star hotel (see p.44)	% percentage rating (see p.44)	♠♣ country house hotel (see p.44)	⌂ travel lodge (see p.43)
GH guest house	**T&C** town & country homes (see p.42)	G1 ground floor bedrooms (A-annexe)	WC toilets *en suite*	access to reception
FH farmhouse	lift	guide dogs	dining room	access to lounge
INN inn	telephone/ intercom	**P** parking at entrance	room service	access to bar

* Details have not been confirmed for 1993. Please check when booking, including information about grab rails.

SOUTH WITHAM New Fox **LINCOLNSHIRE**
LE15 8AU ☎ Thistleton (057283) 586
Central Res (0800) 850950
FORTE TRAVELODGE ⌂
Access through main double doors from car park
via ramp

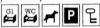

NW3 **CENTRAL LONDON**
128 King Henry's Road Swiss Cottage
☎ 071-722 7711
REGENTS PARK MARRIOTT ★★★★ **65%**
Access through main automatic doors from King
Henry's Road

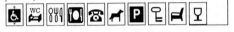

NW3 **CENTRAL LONDON**
2 Fellows Road NW3 3LP ☎ 071-722 5032
SEAFORD LODGE GH
Access through side single door from Fellows
Road

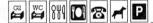

SW1 **CENTRAL LONDON**
Hyde Park Corner SW1X 7TA ☎ 071-259 5599
THE LANESBOROUGH ★★★★★ **84%**
Access through main double doors from
Knightsbridge

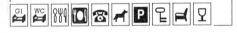

W1 **CENTRAL LONDON**
134 George Street W1H 6DN ☎ 071-723 1277
MARBLE ARCH MARRIOTT ★★★★ **59%**
Access through main single and revolving doors
from George Street via ramp

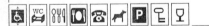

W6 **CENTRAL LONDON**
1 Shortlands W6 8DR ☎ 081-741 1555
NOVOTEL ★★★ **61%**
Access through main double doors from
Shortlands

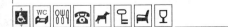

W8 **CENTRAL LONDON**
Scarsdale Place off Wrights Lane W8 5SR
☎ 071-937 7211
LONDON TARA ★★★★ **63%**
Access through main double doors from
Scarsdale Place via ramp

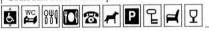

CROYDON 7 Altyre Road **GREATER LONDON**
☎ 081-680 9200
CROYDON PARK ★★★★ **61%**
Access through main automatic doors from Altyre
Road via one step

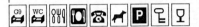

GREENFORD **GREATER LONDON**
Western Avenue UB6 8ST ☎ 081-566 6246
BRIDGE ★★★ **68%**
Access through main double doors from
Greenford Road via ramp

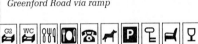

HESTON MOTORWAY **GREATER LONDON**
SERVICE AREA M4 Service Area
North Hyde Lane TW5 9NA ☎ 081-574 5875
GRANADA LODGE ⌂
Access through double doors from car park

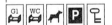

HILLINGDON **GREATER LONDON**
Western Avenue UB10 9NX
☎ Uxbridge (0895) 251199
MASTER BREWER ★★★ **62%**
Access through main single doors from Western
Avenue via one step

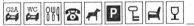

MORDEN Epsom Road **GREATER LONDON**
SM4 5PH ☎ 081-640 8227 Central Res (0800) 850950
FORTE TRAVELODGE ⌂
Access through main double doors from car park
via ramp

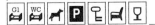

RUISLIP* **GREATER LONDON**
West End Road HA4 6JB ☎ (0895) 636057
BARN GH
Access through main single swing door from West End Road via one step

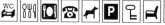

SUTTON **GREATER LONDON**
Gibson Road SM1 2RF ☎ 081-770 1311
HOLIDAY INN ★★★★ 62%
Access through main automatic doors from Gibson Road via ramp

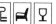

SUTTON* **GREATER LONDON**
135 Cheam Road SM1 2BN ☎ 081-642 3131
THATCHED HOUSE GH
Access through main single door from Cheam Road via one step

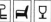

WEST DRAYTON **GREATER LONDON**
Stockley Road UB7 9NA ☎ (0895) 445555
HOLIDAY INN CROWNE PLAZA ★★★★ 59%
Access through revolving and swing doors from Stockley Road via ramp

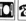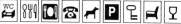

CASTLETOWN Fort Island **ISLE OF MAN**
☎ (0624) 822201
CASTLETOWN GOLF LINKS ★★★ 66%
Access through side double doors

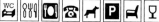

BEBINGTON New Chester Road **MERSEYSIDE**
L62 9AQ ☎ 051-327 2489
Central Res (0800) 850950
FORTE TRAVELODGE ⌂
Access through main double doors from car park via ramp

BROMBOROUGH High Street **MERSEYSIDE**
L62 7HZ ☎ 051-334 2917
CROMWELL ★★★ 67%
Access through double main door from car park via ramp

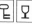

HAYDOCK Lodge Lane **MERSEYSIDE**
Newton−Le−Willows WA12
☎ Wigan (0942) 717878
FORTE POSTHOUSE ★★★ 67%
Access through main double swing doors from Lodge Lane

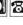

HAYDOCK Piele Road WA11 9TL **MERSEYSIDE**
☎ (0942) 272055 Central Res (0800) 850950
FORTE TRAVELODGE ⌂
Access through main double doors from car park via ramp

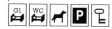

HAYDOCK Penny Lane **MERSEYSIDE**
WA11 9SG ☎ Ashton-in-Makerfield (0942) 272000
HAYDOCK THISTLE ★★★★ 61%
Access through main double doors via ramp

★★★★ hotel rating (see p.43)	**Red Star** highest award to hotel (see p.44)	**%** percentage rating (see p.44)	country house hotel (see p.44)	travel lodge (see p.43)

GH guest house   **T&C** town & country homes (see p.42)   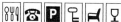 **G1** ground floor bedrooms (A-annexe)   **WC** toilets *en suite*   access to reception

FH farmhouse   lift   guide dogs   dining room   access to lounge

INN inn   ☎ telephone/intercom   **P** parking at entrance   room service   access to bar

* Details have not been confirmed for 1993. Please check when booking, including information about grab rails.

LIVERPOOL Chaloner Street **MERSEYSIDE**
Queens Dock ☎ 051-709 8104
CAMPANILE ⌂
Access through swing doors from car park off
Wapping and Chaloner Street

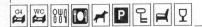

LIVERPOOL* Paradise Street **MERSEYSIDE**
L1 8JD ☎ 051-709 0181
LIVERPOOL MOAT HOUSE ★★★★ 59%
Access through main automatic doors from
Paradise Street via ramp

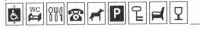

SOUTHPORT* Promenade **MERSEYSIDE**
PR8 1RB ☎ (0704) 533771
ROYAL CLIFTON ★★★ 62%
Access through main double doors from
Promenade

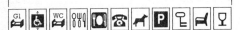

ACLE A47 Acle Bypass **NORFOLK**
☎ (0493) 751970 Central Res (0800) 850950
FORTE TRAVELODGE ⌂
Access through main double doors from car park
via ramp

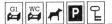

BARNHAM BROOM NR9 4DD **NORFOLK**
☎ (060545) 393
BARNHAM BROOM ★★★ 65%
Access through main double doors from
Honingham Road via one step. No grab rails in
bathroom

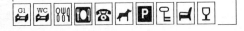

BLAKENEY* NR25 7ND **NORFOLK**
☎ Cley (0263) 740376
MANOR ★★ 61%
Access through single door from car park off The
Quay

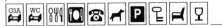

HUNSTANTON **NORFOLK**
Old Hunstanton Road PE36 6HH
☎ (0485) 533486
CALEY HALL ★★ 67%
Access through main double doors via ramp. No
grab rails in bathrooms

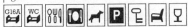

KING'S LYNN* Knights Hill Village **NORFOLK**
South Wootton PE30 3HQ ☎ (0553) 675566
KNIGHTS HILL ★★★ 70%
Access through main double swing doors

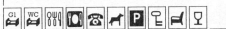

NORWICH 2 Barnard Road **NORFOLK**
NR5 9JB ☎ (0603) 741161
FRIENDLY ★★★ 62%
Access through main double automatic doors
from Barnard Road via ramp

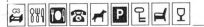

GREAT YARMOUTH Albert Square **NORFOLK**
NR30 3JH
☎ (0493) 855070
MERIDIAN DOLPHIN ★★★ 60%
Access through main double doors from Albert
Square via ramp

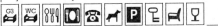

CORBY* **NORTHAMPTONSHIRE**
Rockingham Road NN17 1AE ☎ (0536) 401348
FORTE POSTHOUSE ★★★ 62%
Access through main swing doors from
Rockingham Lane

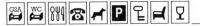

DAVENTRY **NORTHAMPTONSHIRE**
Ashby Road (A361) NN11 5NX ☎ (0327) 301777
DAVENTRY RESORT ★★★ 65%
Access through main double automatic doors via
ramp

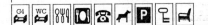

DESBOROUGH **NORTHAMPTONSHIRE**
A6 Harborough Road
☎ (0536) 762034 Central Res (0800) 850950
FORTE TRAVELODGE ⌂
Access through main double doors from car park
via ramp

FLORE **NORTHAMPTONSHIRE**
The High Street NN7 4LP ☎ Weedon (0327) 349022
HEYFORD MANOR ★★★ **64%**
Access through main or rear double swing doors.
Grab rails around toilet only

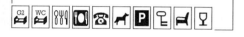

NORTHAMPTON **NORTHAMPTONSHIRE**
Upton Way NN5 6EG
☎ (0604) 758395 Central Res (0800) 850950
FORTE TRAVELODGE ⌂
Access through main double doors from car park
via ramp

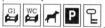

NORTHAMPTON **NORTHAMPTONSHIRE**
Eagle Drive NN4 0HW ☎ (0604) 768700
SWALLOW ★★★★ **59%**
Access through main double doors from Eagle
Drive

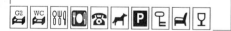

THRAPSTON **NORTHAMPTONSHIRE**
A14 Thrapston Bypass
☎ (0801) 25199 Central Res (0800) 850950
FORTE TRAVELODGE ⌂
Access through main double doors from car park
via ramp

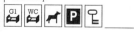

TOWCESTER A43 **NORTHAMPTONSHIRE**
East Towcester Bypass NN12 0DD
☎ (0327) 359105 Central Res (0800) 850950
FORTE TRAVELODGE ⌂
Access through main double doors from car park
via ramp

ALLENDALE NE47 9EJ **NORTHUMBERLAND**
☎ Hexham (0434) 683248
BISHOPFIELD COUNTRY HOUSE ★★ **70%** ♠♣
Access through main single door via two steps.
No grab rails in bathroom

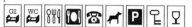

LONGHORSLEY **NORTHUMBERLAND**
NE65 8XF ☎ Morpeth (0670) 516611
LINDEN HALL ★★★★ **75%**
Access through side double doors via ramp.
No grab rails in bathroom

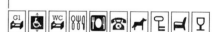

BOLTON ABBEY **NORTH YORKSHIRE**
BD23 6AJ ☎ (0756) 710441
DEVONSHIRE ARMS
COUNTRY HOUSE ★★★ **79%**
Access through main double swing doors via ramp

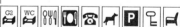

BOROUGHBRIDGE **NORTH YORKSHIRE**
Roecliffe YO5 9LY ☎ (0423) 322578
CROWN INN INN
Access through double doors from car park via
one step. Grab rails around bath only

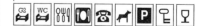

★★★★ hotel rating (see p.43)	★ Red highest award to Star hotel (see p.44)
GH guest house	**T&C** town & country homes (see p.42)
FH farmhouse	lift
INN inn	telephone/intercom

 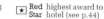 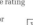 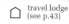 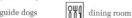   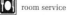

% percentage rating (see p.44)   country house hotel (see p.44)   ⌂ travel lodge (see p.43)

G1 ground floor bedrooms (A-annexe)   WC toilets *en suite*   access to reception

guide dogs   dining room   access to lounge

P parking at entrance   room service   access to bar

* Details have not been confirmed for 1993. Please check when booking, including information about grab rails.

| HARROGATE | NORTH YORKSHIRE |

3-13 Swan Road HG1 2SS ☎ (0423) 560666
GRANTS ★★★ **68%**
Access through main double doors from Swan
Road. Grab rails around toilet only

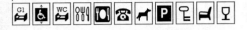

| NORTHALLERTON | NORTH YORKSHIRE |

Darlington Road DL6 2XF ☎ (0609) 780525
SUNDIAL ★★★ **66%**
Access through main double doors from
Darlington Road

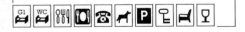

| HARROGATE | NORTH YORKSHIRE |

Kings Road HG1 1XX ☎ (0423) 500000
MOAT HOUSE INTERNATIONAL ★★★★ **64%**
Access through main automatic doors from Kings
Road

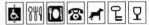

| SCOTCH CORNER | NORTH YORKSHIRE |

Skeeby DL10 5EQ ☎ Richmond (0748) 3768
Central Res (0800) 850950
FORTE TRAVELODGE ⌂
Access through main double doors from car park
via ramp

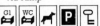

| HELMSLEY Harome | NORTH YORKSHIRE |

YO6 JG ☎ (0439) 71241
PHEASANT ★★ **72%**
Access through main double doors

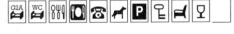

| SCOTCH CORNER | NORTH YORKSHIRE |

A1/A66 Middleton Tyas Lane DL10 6PQ
☎ Darlington (0325) 377177
PAVILION LODGE ⌂
Access through main double doors via ramp

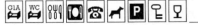

| KETTLEWELL BD23 5RJ | NORTH YORKSHIRE |

☎ (0756) 760243
LANGCLIFFE HOUSE GH
Access through double doors from car park via
ramp

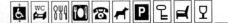

| SKIPTON | NORTH YORKSHIRE |

Gargrave Road BD23 1UD
☎ (0756) 798091 Central Res (0800) 850950
FORTE TRAVELODGE ⌂
Access through main double doors from car park
via ramp

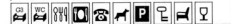

| LEEMING BAR* DL7 9AY | NORTH YORKSHIRE |

☎ Bedale (0677) 422707 & 424941
WHITE ROSE ★★ **61%**
Access through single door from car park via one
step

| WEST WITTON* | NORTH YORKSHIRE |

DL8 4LS ☎ Wensleydale (0969) 22322
WENSLEYDALE HEIFER INN ★★ **68%**
Access through main single door from Main Street
via two steps

| LEYBURN | NORTH YORKSHIRE |

Market Place DL8 5AS ☎ Wensleydale (0969) 22161
GOLDEN LION ★ **58%**
Access through main single door from Market
Square via one step

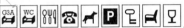

| YORK Water End | NORTH YORKSHIRE |

Clifton YO3 6LL ☎ (0904) 610510
CLIFTON BRIDGE ★★ **63%**
Access through main single door from
Westminster Road. No grab rails in bathroom

YORK Tower Street **NORTH YORKSHIRE**
YO1 1SB ☎ (0904) 648111
HOLIDAY INN ★★★★ **62%**
Access through main automatic doors from Tower
Street via ramp

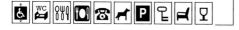

YORK 129 Holgate Road **NORTH YORKSHIRE**
YO2 4DE ☎ (0904) 625787
KILIMA ★★ **74%**
Access through main single door from Holgate
Road via ramp

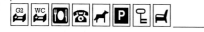

YORK* Fishergate **NORTH YORKSHIRE**
YO1 4AD ☎ (0904) 611660
NOVOTEL ★★★ **63%**
Access through main double electric doors from
Fishergate

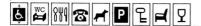

YORK Tadcaster Road **NORTH YORKSHIRE**
YO2 2QQ ☎ (0904) 701000
SWALLOW ★★★★ **64%**
Access through front automatic sliding doors from
Tadcaster Road

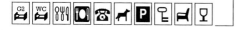

BLYTH A1 (Southbound) **NOTTINGHAMSHIRE**
☎ (0909) 591775 Central Res (0800) 850950
FORTE TRAVELODGE ⌂
Access through main double doors from car park
via ramp

BLYTH **NOTTINGHAMSHIRE**
Hilltop Roundabout S81 8HG (jnct A1M/A614)
☎ (0909) 591836
GRANADA LODGE ⌂
Access through main double doors from car park
off Hilltop Roundabout

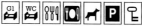

MARKHAM MOOR **NOTTINGHAMSHIRE**
A1 (Northbound) DN22 0QU
☎ Retford (0777) 838091 Central Res (0800) 850950
FORTE TRAVELODGE ⌂
Access through main double doors from car park
via ramp

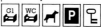

NEWARK-ON-TRENT **NOTTINGHAMSHIRE**
North Muskham (3m N on A1) NG23 6HT
☎ (0636) 703635 Central Res (0800) 850950
FORTE TRAVELODGE ⌂
Access through main double doors from car park
via ramp

NOTTINGHAM **NOTTINGHAMSHIRE**
Castle Marina Park NG7 1GX ☎ (0602) 500600
HOLIDAY INN GARDEN COURT ★★★ **58%**
Access through main double doors from Castle
Marina Park via ramp

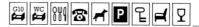

NOTTINGHAM **NOTTINGHAMSHIRE**
Mansfield Road NG5 2BT ☎ (0602) 602621
NOTTINGHAM MOAT HOUSE ★★★ **69%**
Access through rear double doors from Zulla
Road

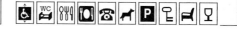

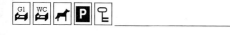

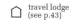

★★★★ hotel rating (see p.43)	⊠ Red Star highest award to hotel (see p.44)	% percentage rating (see p.44)	� country house hotel (see p.44)	⌂ travel lodge (see p.43)
GH guest house	**T&C** town & country homes (see p.42)	G1 🛏 ground floor bedrooms (A-annexe)	WC 🛏 toilets *en suite*	⌴ access to reception
FH farmhouse	🦽 lift	🐕 guide dogs	dining room	access to lounge
INN inn	☎ telephone/ intercom	P parking at entrance	room service	access to bar

* Details have not been confirmed for 1993. Please check when booking, including information about grab rails.

75

NOTTINGHAM **NOTTINGHAMSHIRE**
Wollaton Street NG1 5RH ☎ (0602) 414444
ROYAL MOAT HOUSE
INTERNATIONAL ★★★★ 64%
Access through main single door from Wollaton
Street via ramp

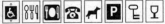

NOTTINGHAM* **NOTTINGHAMSHIRE**
Milton Street NG1 3PZ ☎ (0602) 419561
STAKIS VICTORIA ★★★ 59%
Access through main swing door from Milton
Street via ramp

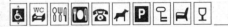

WORKSOP **NOTTINGHAMSHIRE**
Clumber Park S80 3PA
☎ Mansfield (0623) 835333
CLUMBER PARK ★★★ 69%
Access through level double doors

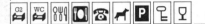

ABINGDON Marcham Road **OXFORDSHIRE**
OX14 1TZ ☎ (0235) 553456
ABINGDON LODGE ★★★ 62%
Access through main double swing door via ramp

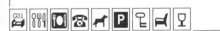

GREAT MILTON OX44 7PD **OXFORDSHIRE**
☎ (0844) 278881
LE MANOIR
AUX QUAT' SAISONS ★★★★ Red ♨
Access through main single door from Church
Road. No grab rails in bathroom

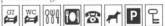

LEW University Farm **OXFORDSHIRE**
OX18 2AU ☎ Bampton Castle (0993) 850297
FARMHOUSE HOTEL & RESTAURANT FH
Access through main single door

OXFORD* Godstow Road **OXFORDSHIRE**
OX2 8AL ☎ (0865) 59933
OXFORD MOAT HOUSE ★★★ 64%
Access through main double doors from Linton
Road via one step

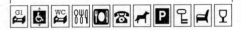

OXFORD **OXFORDSHIRE**
Hinksey Hill Top OX1 5BG ☎ (0865) 735408
WESTWOOD COUNTRY HOTEL GH
Access through side single door from Hinksey Hill

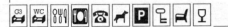

WHEATLEY **OXFORDSHIRE**
London Road (off A40)
☎ (0867) 75705 Central Res (0800) 850950
FORTE TRAVELODGE ⌂
Access through main double doors from car park
via ramp

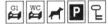

MARKET DRAYTON* **SHROPSHIRE**
Goldstone TF9 2NA
☎ Cheswardine (063086) 202 & 487
GOLDSTONE HALL ★★★ 70%
Access through main single door from Goldstone
Road

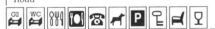

OSWESTRY **SHROPSHIRE**
Mile End Service Area SY11 4JA (jnct A5/A483)
☎ (0691) 658178 Central Res (0800) 850950
TRAVELODGE ⌂
Access through main double doors from car park
via ramp

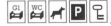

TELFORD St Quentin Gate **SHROPSHIRE**
TF3 4EH ☎ (0952) 292500
HOLIDAY INN ★★★ 69%
Access through main automatic doors from car
park off St Quentin Gate

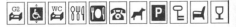

TELFORD Forgegate | **SHROPSHIRE**
Telford Centre TF3 4NA ☎ (0952) 291291
TELFORD MOAT HOUSE ★★★ 69%
Access through main swing doors from Forgegate via ramp

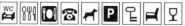

WHITCHURCH Hill Valley | **SHROPSHIRE**
SY13 4JZ ☎ (0948) 3031
TERRICK HALL COUNTRY ★★★ 63%
Access through main single door from Terrick Road via two steps. No grab rails in bathroom

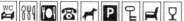

WORFIELD WV15 5JZ | **SHROPSHIRE**
☎ (07464) 497
OLD VICARAGE ★★★ 72%
Access through main single door via ramp. Grab rails around toilet only

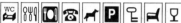

BRIDGWATER 37 St Mary Street | **SOMERSET**
TA6 3LX ☎ (0278) 452859
FRIARN COURT ★★ 64%
Access through rear single door via ramp. No grab rails in bathroom

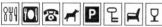

BRIDGWATER North Petherton | **SOMERSET**
TA6 6QA ☎ North Petherton (0278) 662255
WALNUT TREE INN ★★★ 70%
Access through main single door. Grab rails around bath only

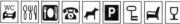

DULVERTON TA22 9AE | **SOMERSET**
☎ (0398) 23302
CARNARVON ARMS ★★★ 71% ⚘
Access through main double doors via ramp

ILMINSTER A303 | **SOMERSET**
☎ (0460) 53748 Central Res (0800) 850950
FORTE TRAVELODGE ⌂
Access through main double doors from car park via ramp

    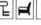

ILMINSTER TA19 9AR | **SOMERSET**
☎ (0460) 52108
SHRUBBERY ★★ 62%
Access through main double door from Station Road via one step. Grab rails around baths only

MINEHEAD Northfield Road | **SOMERSET**
TA24 5PU ☎ (0643) 705155
NORTHFIELD ★★★ 67%
Access through main single door from Northfield Road. Grab rails around toilet only

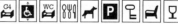

MINEHEAD The Esplanade | **SOMERSET**
☎ (0643) 702572
PROMENADE
Access through main single door (Run by John Grooms Association)

★★★★	hotel rating (see p.43)	★ Red Star	highest award to hotel (see p.44)	%	percentage rating (see p.44)	⚘	country house hotel (see p.44)	⌂	travel lodge (see p.43)
GH	guest house	**T&C**	town & country homes (see p.42)	G1	ground floor bedrooms (A-annexe)	WC	toilets *en suite*		access to reception
FH	farmhouse		lift		guide dogs		dining room		access to lounge
INN	inn	☎	telephone/ intercom	P	parking at entrance		room service	♀	access to bar

* Details have not been confirmed for 1993. Please check when booking, including information about grab rails.

MUDFORD Main Street BA21 5TF **SOMERSET**
☎ Marston Magna (0935) 850289
HALF MOON INN INN
Access through side single door from Main Street
via ramp

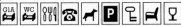

PODIMORE BA22 8JG **SOMERSET**
☎ Yeovil (0935) 840074 Central Res (0800) 850950
FORTE TRAVELODGE ⌂
Access through main double doors from car park
via ramp

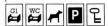

SEDGEMOOR MOTORWAY **SOMERSET**
SERVICE AREA (M5) M5 Motorway Northbound
BS24 0JL ☎ (0934) 750831 Central Res (0800) 850950
FORTE TRAVELODGE ⌂
Access through main double doors from car park
via ramp

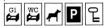

TAUNTON Rumwell TA4 1EL **SOMERSET**
☎ (0823) 461902
RUMWELL MANOR ★★★ **66%**
Access through rear single door from Wallington
Road

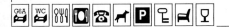

TAUNTON DEANE MOTORWAY **SOMERSET**
SERVICE AREA Trull TA1 4BA
☎ Taunton (0823) 332228
ROADCHEF LODGE ⌂
Access through main double doors

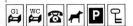

BARNSLEY A633/635 **SOUTH YORKSHIRE**
Stairfoot Roundabout
☎ (0226) 298799 Central Res (0800) 850950
FORTE TRAVELODGE ⌂
Access through main double doors from car park
via ramp

CARCROFT A1 **SOUTH YORKSHIRE**
Great North Road ☎
(0302) 330841 Central Res (0800) 850950
FORTE TRAVELODGE ⌂
Access through main double doors from car park
via ramp

DONCASTER **SOUTH YORKSHIRE**
Doncaster Leisure Park Bantry Road DN4 7PD
☎ (0302) 370770
CAMPANILE ⌂
Access through main single door from Bantry
Road via ramp

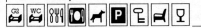

DONCASTER **SOUTH YORKSHIRE**
Warmsworth DN4 9UX ☎ (0302) 310331
DONCASTER MOAT HOUSE ★★★ **67%**
Access through main double doors from Sheffield
Road via ramp

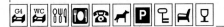

HOOTON ROBERTS* **SOUTH YORKSHIRE**
S65 4PF ☎ Rotherham (0709) 852737
EARL OF STRAFFORD ★★ **70%**
Access through main double doors

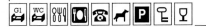

ROSSINGTON **SOUTH YORKSHIRE**
Great North Road DN11 0HP
☎ Doncaster (0302) 868219
MOUNT PLEASANT ★★★ **64%**
Access through main double doors from Great
North Road

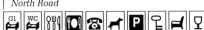

ROTHERHAM* **SOUTH YORKSHIRE**
Moorgate Road S60 2TY ☎ (0709) 382772
BRENTWOOD ★★ **69%**
Access through front double door (via rear car
park) from Moorgate Road via two steps

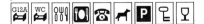

ROTHERHAM	SOUTH YORKSHIRE

Hellaby Industrial Estate Lowton Way
off Denby Way S66 8RY ☎ (0709) 700255
CAMPANILE ⌂
Access through main single door from Lowton
Way via ramp

THURCROFT*	SOUTH YORKSHIRE

Brampton Road S66 9JA
☎ Rotherham (0709) 530022
CONSORT ★★★ **65%**
Access through main double doors from
Brampton Road via one step

SHEFFIELD	SOUTH YORKSHIRE

161 Abbeydale Road S7 2QW ☎ (0742) 620500
BEAUCHIEF ★★★ **68%**
Access through swing doors from car park off
Abbey Lane. No grab rails in bathroom

TODWICK Worksop Road	SOUTH YORKSHIRE

S31 0DJ ☎ Worksop (0909) 771654
RED LION ★★★ **68%**
Access through main double swing door

SHEFFIELD	SOUTH YORKSHIRE

340 Prince of Wales Road S2 1FF ☎ (0742)
530935
GRANADA ★★★ **60%**
Access through main double doors from Prince of
Wales Road via ramp

BARTON-UNDER-	STAFFORDSHIRE

NEEDWOOD (on A38, northbound)
☎ (0283) 716343 Central Res (0800) 850950
FORTE TRAVELODGE ⌂
Access through main double doors from car park
via ramp

SHEFFIELD	SOUTH YORKSHIRE

Chesterfield Road South S8 8BW ☎ (0742) 375376
SHEFFIELD MOAT HOUSE ★★★ **71%**
Access through main electric doors from
Chesterfield Road South

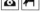

BARTON-UNDER-	STAFFORDSHIRE

NEEDWOOD Rykneld Street (on A38, southbound)
☎ (0283) 716784 Central Res (0800) 850950
FORTE TRAVELODGE ⌂
Access through main double doors from car park
via ramp

THORNE Horsefair Green	SOUTH YORKSHIRE

DN8 5EE ☎ (0405) 812320
BELMONT ★★ **67%**
Access through double doors from car park via
ramp. No grab rails in bathroom

RUGELEY	STAFFORDSHIRE

Western Springs Road WS15 2AS (A51)
☎ (0889) 570096 Central Res (0800) 850950
FORTE TRAVELODGE ⌂
Access through main double doors from car park
via ramp

★★★★ hotel rating (see p.43)	★ Red Star highest award to hotel (see p.44)	% percentage rating (see p.44)	♣♣ country house hotel (see p.44)	⌂ travel lodge (see p.43)
GH guest house	**T&C** town & country homes (see p.42)	G1 ground floor bedrooms (A-annexe)	WC toilets *en suite*	access to reception
FH farmhouse	lift	guide dogs	dining room	access to lounge
INN inn	telephone/ intercom	**P** parking at entrance	room service	access to bar

* Details have not been confirmed for 1993. Please check when booking, including information about grab rails.

STOKE-ON-TRENT **STAFFORDSHIRE**
Etruria Hall Festival Way ST1 5BQ
☎ (0782) 219000
STOKE-ON-TRENT MOAT HOUSE ★★★★ **62%**
Access through main electric door from Festival
Way

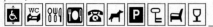

STONE ST15 0BQ **STAFFORDSHIRE**
☎ (0785) 815531
STONE HOUSE ★★★ **67%**
Access through main double doors.
Grab rails around bath only

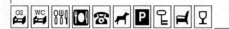

TAMWORTH B77 5PS **STAFFORDSHIRE**
(A5/M42 jnct 10) ☎ (0827) 260123
GRANADA LODGE ⌂
Access through main double doors from car park

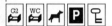

UTTOXETER **STAFFORDSHIRE**
Ashbourne Road ST14 5AA
☎ (0889) 562043 Central Res (0800) 850950
FORTE TRAVELODGE ⌂
Access through main double doors from car park
via ramp

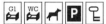

ALDEBURGH Victoria Road **SUFFOLK**
IP15 5DX ☎ (0728) 452420
UPLANDS ★★ **65%**
Access through main double doors from Victoria
Road

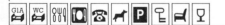

BARTON MILLS IP28 6AE (A11) **SUFFOLK**
☎ (0638) 717675 Central Res (0800) 850950
FORTE TRAVELODGE ⌂
Access through main double doors from car park
via ramp

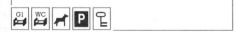

HADLEIGH 131 High Street IP7 5EJ **SUFFOLK**
☎ Ipswich (0473) 822032
ODDS & ENDS GH
Access through side door from High Street.
Grab rails around toilet only

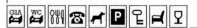

IPSWICH Belstead Road IP2 9HB **SUFFOLK**
☎ (0473) 68424
BELSTEAD BROOK ★★★ **72%**
Access through main double doors from Belstead
Road

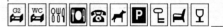

IPSWICH London Road Copdock **SUFFOLK**
IP8 3JD ☎ (0473) 730444
IPSWICH MOAT HOUSE ★★★ **65%**
Access through main double doors from Old
London Road via ramp

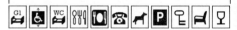

IPSWICH Henley Road IP1 3SP **SUFFOLK**
☎ (0473) 257677
MARLBOROUGH ★★★ **70%**
Access through main double doors from Henley
Road via ramp

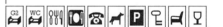

IPSWICH The Haven **SUFFOLK**
Ransomes Europark IP3 9SJ ☎ (0473) 272244
SUFFOLK GRANGE ★★★ **71%**
Access through main double swing doors from the
Havens via ramp

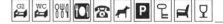

MILDENHALL* Beck Row IP28 8DH **SUFFOLK**
☎ (0638) 713223
SMOKE HOUSE INN ★★★ **65%**
Access through main swing doors via ramp

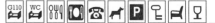

NEWMARKET Moulton Road **SUFFOLK**
CB8 8DY ☎ (0638) 667171
NEWMARKET MOAT HOUSE ★★★ **65%**
Access through main double doors from Moulton
Road via one step. Grab rails around bath only

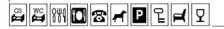

NUTFIELD RH1 4EN **SURREY**
☎ Redhill (0737) 822066
NUTFIELD PRIORY ★★★ **74%**
Access through double front door via ramp.
No grab rails in bathroom

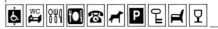

STOWMARKET IP14 3PY (A45) **SUFFOLK**
☎ (0449) 615347 Central Res (0800) 850950
FORTE TRAVELODGE ⌂
Access through main double doors from car park
via ramp

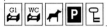

FELLING Leam Lane Wardley **TYNE & WEAR**
Whitemare Pool NE10 8YB
☎ 091-438 3333 Central Res (0800) 850950
FORTE TRAVELODGE ⌂
Access through main double doors from car
parking via ramp

BURGH HEATH* Brighton Road **SURREY**
KT20 6BW ☎ (0737) 353355
HEATHSIDE HOTEL ★★ **62%**
Access through main doors from Brighton Road

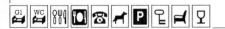

NEWCASTLE UPON TYNE **TYNE & WEAR**
New Bridge Street NE1 8BS ☎ 091-232 6191
FORTE CREST ★★★ **66%**
Access through main double doors from New
Bridge Street

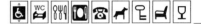

DORKING Reigate Road **SURREY**
RH4 1QB (A25)
☎ (0306) 740361 Central Res (0800) 850950
FORTE TRAVELODGE ⌂
Access through main double doors from car park
via ramp

SEATON BURN **TYNE & WEAR**
Great North Road NE13 6BP ☎ 091-236 5432
HOLIDAY INN NEWCASTLE ★★★★ **54%**
Access through main double doors from Great
North Road via ramp

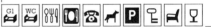

GUILDFORD Egerton Road GU2 5XZ **SURREY**
☎ (0483) 574444
FORTE CREST ★★★★ **62%**
Access through main double swing doors from
Egerton Road via ramp

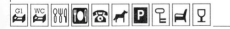

SUNDERLAND **TYNE & WEAR**
Queen's Parade SR6 8DB ☎ 091-529 2041
SWALLOW ★★★ **72%**
Access through main double swing doors from car
park via ramp

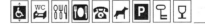

★★★★	hotel rating (see p.43)	★ Red Star	highest award to hotel (see p.44)	%	percentage rating (see p.44)	♣ country house hotel (see p.44)	⌂ travel lodge (see p.43)
GH guest house		**T&C** town & country homes (see p.42)	G1 ground floor bedrooms (A-annexe)	WC toilets *en suite*	access to reception
FH farmhouse		lift	guide dogs	dining room	access to lounge
INN inn		telephone/intercom	P parking at entrance	room service	access to bar

* **Details have not been confirmed for 1993. Please check when booking, including information about grab rails.**

WASHINGTON SERVICE
AREA* Portobello (A1M) ☎ 091-410 0076
GRANADA LODGE ⌂
Access through double doors from car park via ramp

TYNE & WEAR

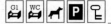

WHICKHAM Front Street
NE16 4JG ☎ 091-488 8000
GIBSIDE ARMS ★★★ 71%
Access through rear double doors from Front Street via one step

TYNE & WEAR

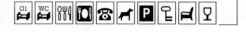

WHITLEY BAY*
160-164 Park Avenue NE26 1AU ☎ 091-253 0288
PARK LODGE ★★ 60%
Access through side and rear single doors from Park Avenue via one step

TYNE & WEAR

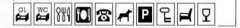

CHARLECOTE CV35 9EW
☎ (0789) 470333
CHARLECOTE PHEASANT COUNTRY ★★★ 58%
Access through main double swing doors via ramp

WARWICKSHIRE

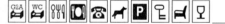

HONILEY CV8 1NP
☎ Kenilworth (0926) 484234
HONILEY COURT ★★★ 66%
Access through main double swing door via ramp

WARWICKSHIRE

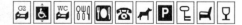

NUNEATON
Bedworth CV12 0BN (A444)
☎ (0203) 382541 Central Res (0800) 850950
FORTE TRAVELODGE ⌂
Access through main double doors from car park via ramp

WARWICKSHIRE

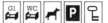

SIBSON Main Road
CV13 6LB ☎ Tamworth (0827) 880223
MILLERS ★★ 65%
Access through main double swing doors from Main Road via ramp. Grab rails around bath only

WARWICKSHIRE

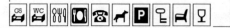

STRATFORD-UPON-AVON
Bridgefoot CV37 6YR ☎ (0789) 414411
MOAT HOUSE INTERNATIONAL ★★★★ 62%
Access through main single door from Bridgefoot via ramp

WARWICKSHIRE

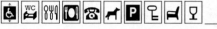

STRATFORD-UPON-AVON
Warwick Road CV37 0NR ☎ (0789) 295252
**WELCOMBE HOTEL
& GOLF COURSE** ★★★★ 64%
Access through main double doors from Warwick Road via two steps

WARWICKSHIRE

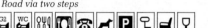

THURLASTON London Road
CV23 9LG (A45) ☎ Dunchurch (0788) 521538
Central Res (0800) 850950
FORTE TRAVELODGE ⌂
Access through main double doors from car park via ramp

WARWICKSHIRE

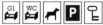

BIRMINGHAM
55 Irving Street B1 1Dh ☎ 021-622 4925
CAMPANILE ⌂
Access through main single swing door via ramp

WEST MIDLANDS

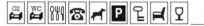

BIRMINGHAM
Holliday Street B1 1HH ☎ 021-631 2000
HOLIDAY INN ★★★★ 58%
Access through main automatic doors via ramp. No grab rails in bathroom

WEST MIDLANDS

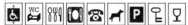

BIRMINGHAM AIRPORT | **WEST MIDLANDS**
B26 3QL ☎ 021-782 7000
NOVOTEL ★★★ **61%**
Access through main double automatic doors
from Novotel Way

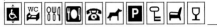

COVENTRY Holyhead Road | **WEST MIDLANDS**
CV5 8HX ☎ (0203) 601601
BROOKLANDS GARAGE ★★★ **68%**
Access through main double swing doors from car
park off Holyhead Road via ramp. No grab rails in
private bathrooms

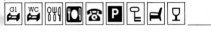

COVENTRY | **WEST MIDLANDS**
Abbey Road Whitley CV3 4BJ ☎ (0203) 639922
CAMPANILE ⌂
Access through single door from car park off
Abbey Road via ramp

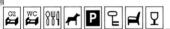

COVENTRY | **WEST MIDLANDS**
Ryton on Dunsmore CV8 3DY ☎ (0203) 301585
COVENTRY KNIGHT ★★★ **66%**
Access through main automatic doors from
London Road. No grab rails in bathroom

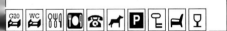

COVENTRY* | **WEST MIDLANDS**
Hinckley Road Walsgrave CV2 2HP
☎ (0203) 613261
FORTE CREST ★★★ **63%**
Access through main electronic double doors
from Hinckley Road via ramp

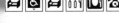
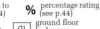

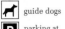

DUDLEY Dudley Road (A461) | **WEST MIDLANDS**
☎ (0384) 481579 Central Res (0800) 850950
FORTE TRAVELODGE ⌂
Access through main double doors from car park
via ramp

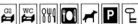

FRANKLEY MOTORWAY | **WEST MIDLANDS**
SERVICE AREA Illey Lane B32 4AR
☎ 021-550 3261
GRANADA LODGE ⌂
Access through main double doors

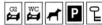

HILTON PARK | **WEST MIDLANDS**
MOTORWAY SERVICE AREA
Hilton Park Services (M6), Essington WV11 2DR
☎ Cheslyn Hay (0922) 414100
PAVILION LODGE ⌂
Access through double doors from car park

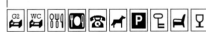

MERIDEN CV7 7NH | **WEST MIDLANDS**
☎ (0676) 22735
MANOR ★★★ **68%**
Access through rear double doors from car park
off Main Road via ramp

OLDBURY | **WEST MIDLANDS**
Wolverhampton Road B69 2BH
☎ 021-552 2967 Central Res (0800) 850950
FORTE TRAVELODGE ⌂
Access through main double doors from car park
via ramp

SOLIHULL | **WEST MIDLANDS**

651 Warwick Road B91 1AT ☎ 021-711 3000
ST JOHN'S SWALLOW ★★★ 64%
Access through main double swing doors from
Warwick Road via ramp

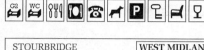

STOURBRIDGE | **WEST MIDLANDS**

260 Hagley Road DY9 0RW
☎ Hagley (0562) 882689
LIMES GH
Access through main double doors from Hagley
Road via two steps

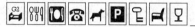

WALSALL Bescot Road | **WEST MIDLANDS**

WS2 9AD ☎ (0922) 27413
ABBERLEY ★★ 65%
Access through rear double doors from car park
via ramp. Grab rails around toilet only

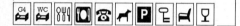

WALSALL 20 Wolverhampton | **WEST MIDLANDS**

Road West WS2 0BS ☎ (0922) 724444
FRIENDLY ★★★ 66%
Access through main automatic doors from
Wolverhampton Road West. Grab rails around
bath only

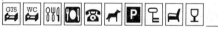

COPTHORNE* | **WEST SUSSEX**

West Park Road R10 3EU ☎ (0342) 714994
COPTHORNE EFFINGHAM PARK ★★★★ 66%
Access through main automatic double doors
from West Park Road via one step

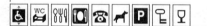

FIVE OAKS RH14 9AE | **WEST SUSSEX**

(on A29) ☎ Billingshurst (0403) 782711
Central Res (0800) 850950
FORTE TRAVELODGE ⌂
Access through main double doors from car park
via ramp

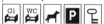

FONTWELL BN18 0SB | **WEST SUSSEX**

(on A27) ☎ Eastergate (0243) 543973
Central Res (0800) 850950
FORTE TRAVELODGE ⌂
Access through main double doors from car park
via ramp

GOODWOOD PO18 0QB | **WEST SUSSEX**

☎ Chichester (0243) 775537
GOODWOOD PARK ★★★ 66%
Access through main double swing doors from
Waterbeach via one step

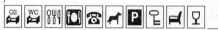

LOWER BEEDING | **WEST SUSSEX**

Brighton Road RH13 6PS ☎ (0403) 891711
SOUTH LODGE ★★★★ 72% ♠
Access through main double doors via ramp.
No grab rails in bathroom

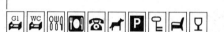

WORTHING | **WEST SUSSEX**

14/20 Windsor Road BN11 2LX ☎ (0903) 239655
WINDSOR HOUSE ★★ 64%
Access through main double swing doors from
Windsor Road

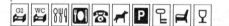

BATLEY* | **WEST YORKSHIRE**

Towngate Road off Healey Lane WF17 7HR
☎ (0924) 444777
ALDER HOUSE ★★ 66%
Access through double swing doors from car park
off Towngate Road via ramp

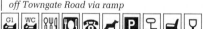   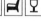

BRADFORD* | **WEST YORKSHIRE**

Merrydale Road ☎ (0274) 683683
NOVOTEL ★★★ 57%
Access through main double swing doors from
Merrydale Road via ramp

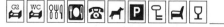

BRADFORD **WEST YORKSHIRE**
Frizinghall BD9 4JY ☎ (0274) 543444
PARK GROVE ★ 69%
Access through single door from car park off Park
Grove via one step. No grab rails in bathroom

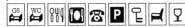

FERRYBRIDGE SERVICE **WEST YORKSHIRE**
AREA WF11 0AF (A1/M62 jnct 33)
☎ Knottingley (0977) 670488
GRANADA LODGE ○
Access through main double swing doors via
ramp

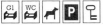

HAREWOOD **WEST YORKSHIRE**
Harrogate Road LS17 9LH ☎ (0532) 886566
HAREWOOD ARMS ★★★ 66%
Access through main single door from Harrogate
Road via two steps. Grab rails around bath only

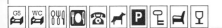

WAKEFIELD **WEST YORKSHIRE**
Denby Dale Road Calder Grove WF4 3QZ
☎ (0924) 276310
CEDAR COURT ★★★ 66%
Access through main automatic sliding doors
from Denby Dale Road via ramp

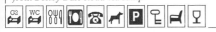

WENTBRIDGE WF8 3JB **WEST YORKSHIRE**
☎ Pontefract (0977) 620711
Central Res (0800) 850950
FORTE TRAVELODGE ○
Access through main double doors from car park
via ramp

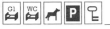

WETHERBY* **WEST YORKSHIRE**
Trip Lane Linton LS22 4JA ☎ (0937) 587271
WOOD HALL ★★★ Red ♣♠
Access through side single door

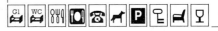

WOOLLEY EDGE **WEST YORKSHIRE**
MOTORWAY SERVICE AREA* M1 Service Area
West Bretton WF4 4LQ ☎ (0924) 830569
GRANADA LODGE ○
Access through main double doors from Bramley
Lane via ramp

SHANKLIN **ISLE OF WIGHT**
Luccombe Road PO37 6RL ☎ (0983) 862719
LUCCOMBE HALL ★★ 64%
Access through large front door.
No grab rails in bathroom

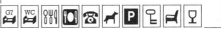

AMESBURY SP4 7AS (on A303) **WILTSHIRE**
☎ (0980) 624966 Central Res (0800) 850950
FORTE TRAVELODGE ○
Access through main double doors from car park
via ramp

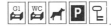

CASTLE COMBE SN14 7HR **WILTSHIRE**
☎ (0249) 782206
MANOR HOUSE ★★★★ 78% ♣♠
Access through main double doors

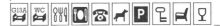

★★★★	hotel rating (see p.43)	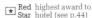 ★ Red Star	highest award to hotel (see p.44)	**%** percentage rating (see p.44)

★★★★ hotel rating (see p.43)　　★ Red Star highest award to hotel (see p.44)　　% percentage rating (see p.44)　　♣♠ country house hotel (see p.44)　　○ travel lodge (see p.43)

GH guest house　　**T&C** town & country homes (see p.42)　　G1 ground floor bedrooms (A-annexe)　　WC toilets *en suite*　　access to reception

FH farmhouse　　♿ lift　　guide dogs　　dining room　　access to lounge

INN inn　　telephone/ intercom　　P parking at entrance　　room service　　access to bar

* Details have not been confirmed for 1993. Please check when booking, including information about grab rails.

LEIGH DELAMERE MOTORWAY **WILTSHIRE**
SERVICE AREA M4 Service Area SN14 6LB
☏ Chippenham (0666) 837097
GRANADA LODGE ⌂
Access through main double doors via ramp

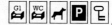

SWINDON Oxford Road **WILTSHIRE**
Stratton St Margaret SN3 4TL ☏ (0793) 831333
FORTE CREST ★★★ **62%**
*Access through main automatic doors from
Oxford Road via ramp*

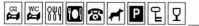

MELKSHAM Beanacre SN12 7PU **WILTSHIRE**
☏ (0225) 703700
BEECHFIELD HOUSE ★★★ **74%** ♿
*Access through front double doors from Beanacre
Road via ramp*

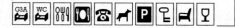

SWINDON Pipers Way SN3 1SH **WILTSHIRE**
☏ (0793) 512121
SWINDON MARRIOTT ★★★★ **61%**
*Access through automatic doors from Pipers Way
via ramp*

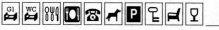

SALISBURY Harnham Road **WILTSHIRE**
Harnham SP2 8JQ ☏ (0722) 327908
ROSE & CROWN ★★★ **66%**
*Access through single and double swing doors
from car park off Harnham Road via ramp*

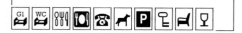

WARMINSTER A36 Bath Road **WILTSHIRE**
BA12 7RU ☏ (0985) 219539
GRANADA LODGE ⌂
*Access through main double swing doors from
Bath Road via ramp*

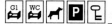

SWINDON Blunsdon SN2 4AD **WILTSHIRE**
(3m N off A419) ☏ (0793) 721701
**BLUNSDON HOUSE HOTEL
& LEISURE CLUB** ★★★★ **73%**
Access through main automatic doors

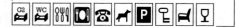

WOOTTON BASSETT **WILTSHIRE**
Coped Hall SN4 8ER ☏ Swindon (0793) 848044
MARSH FARM ★★★ **66%**
*Access through main single door.
Grab rails in bathroom round bath but not toilet*

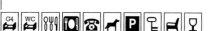

CHANNEL ISLANDS

ST HELIER The Esplanade JE4 8WD **JERSEY**
☏ (0534) 22301
THE GRAND ★★★★ **64%**
*Access through main swing and revolving doors
from The Esplanade via ramp*

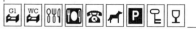

ST SAVIOUR JE2 7SA **JERSEY**
☏ (0534) 25501
LONGUEVILLE MANOR ★★★★ Red ♿
*Access through main double doors from
Longueville Road*

WALES

COLWYN BAY College Avenue **CLWYD**
Rhos-on-Sea LL28 4NT ☎ (0492) 544502
ASHMOUNT ★★ **65%**
Access through side single door from College
Avenue via ramp

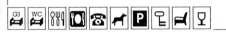

ST ASAPH The Roe LL17 0LT **CLWYD**
☎ (0745) 582263
PLAS ELWY HOTEL & RESTAURANT ★★ **66%**
Access through main single door from The Roe
via two steps. No grab rails in bathroom

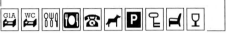

HALKYN CH8 8RF (on A55) **CLWYD**
☎ (0352) 780952 Central Res (0800) 850950
FORTE TRAVELODGE ⌂
Access through main double doors from car park
via ramp

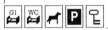

WREXHAM Wrexham By Pass **CLWYD**
Rhostyllen LL14 4EJ
☎ (0978) 365705 Central Res (0800) 850950
FORTE TRAVELODGE ⌂
Access through main double doors from car park
via ramp

NORTHOP HALL CH7 6HB (A55) **CLWYD**
☎ (0244) 816473 Central Res (0800) 850950
FORTE TRAVELODGE ⌂
Access through main double doors from car park
via ramp

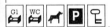

CROSS HANDS SA14 6NW (A48) **DYFED**
☎ (0269) 845700 Central Res (0800) 850950
FORTE TRAVELODGE ⌂
Access through main double doors from car park
via ramp

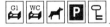

ROSSETT LL12 0AY **CLWYD**
☎ Chester (0244) 571648
LLYNDIR HALL ★★★ **73%**
Access through side single door by leisure club
via ramp

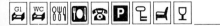

LAMPHEY SA71 5NR **DYFED**
☎ (0646) 672394
LAMPHEY HALL ★★ **69%**
Access through main single door from Upper
Lamphey Road via ramp. Grab rails around bath
only

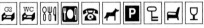
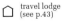

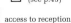
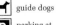

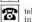
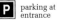

LLANRHYSTUD* SY23 5BZ `DYFED`
☎ Nebo (0974) 272622
PEN-Y-CASTELL FH
Access through side single door from car park via
ramp

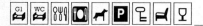

MONMOUTH Cinderhill Street `GWENT`
NP5 3EY ☎ (0600) 715577
RIVERSIDE ★★ **70%**
Access through front and rear, single and double
swing doors via ramp. No grab rails in bathroom

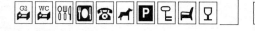

NEWPORT Magor Service Area `GWENT`
(M4 jnct 23) NP6 3YL ☎ Magor (0633) 880111
GRANADA LODGE ⌂
Access through main automatic doors

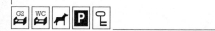

NEWPORT Chepstow Road `GWENT`
Langstone NP6 2LX ☎ (0633) 413737
STAKIS CARDIFF-NEWPORT
COUNTRY COURT ★★★★ **65%**
Access through main double doors from
Chepstow Road

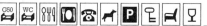

TINTERN NP6 6SF ☎ (0291) 689205 `GWENT`
ROYAL GEORGE ★★ **64%**
Access through main single swing and double
swing doors from car park via one step.
No grab rails in bathroom

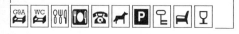

ABERSOCH* Bwlch Tocyn `GWENT`
LL53 7BU ☎ (0758) 713303
PORTH TOCYN ★★★ **65%** ♨
Access through main single door via one step

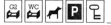

BETWS-Y-COED LL24 0AS `GWYNEDD`
☎ (0690) 710293
CRAIG-Y-DDERWEN
COUNTRY HOUSE ★★★ **64%** ♨
Access through main single door.
Grab rails around shower only

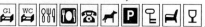

BETWS-Y-COED LL24 0SG `GWYNEDD`
☎ (0690) 710383 & 710787
TY GWYN ★★ **67%**
Access through main single door.
No grab rails in bathroom

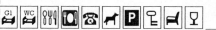

CRICCIETH High Street LL52 0RP `GWYNEDD`
☎ (0766) 522368
PARCIAU MAWR ★★ **66%**
Access through main single door from High Street
via one step

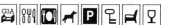

DOLGELLAU Penmaenpool `GWYNEDD`
LL40 1YD ☎ (0341) 422525
GEORGE III ★★ **65%**
Access through main single door from car park.
No grab rails in bathroom

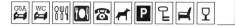

DOLGELLAU Queens Square `GWYNEDD`
LL40 1AR ☎ (0341) 422209
ROYAL SHIP ★★ **63%**
Access through double door from car park off
Queens Square via one step. No grab rails in
bathroom

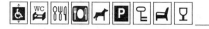

LLANDEGAI Bangor Services `GWYNEDD`
LL57 4BG ☎ Bangor (0248) 370345
PAVILION LODGE ⌂
Access through main automatic double doors

LLANDUDNO* North Parade **GWYNEDD**
LL30 2LP ☎ (0492) 876511
MIN-Y-DON ⭐ **62%**
Access through main double doors from North
Parade

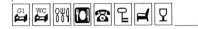

LLANDUDNO* Church Walks **GWYNEDD**
☎ (0492) 76476
ROYAL ⭐⭐ **63%**
Access through double doors from Church Walks

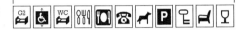

LLANDUDNO West Parade **GWYNEDD**
☎ (0492) 876833
WEST SHORE
Access through main double and single automatic
doors via ramp (Run by John Grooms Association)

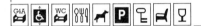

LLANGEFNI* Capel Coch **GWYNEDD**
LL77 7UR ☎ (0248) 750750
TRE-YSGAWEN HALL ⭐⭐⭐ Red ♣
Access through single door from car park

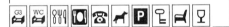

BRIDGEND Ewenny **MID GLAMORGAN**
CF35 5AW ☎ (0656) 668811
HERONSTON ⭐⭐⭐ **65%**
Access through main double and single doors via
ramp. No grab rails in bathroom

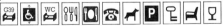

MERTHYR TYDFIL **MID GLAMORGAN**
Park Terrace CF47 8RF ☎ (0685) 723627 & 382055
TREGENNA ⭐⭐ **67%**
Access through single swing doors from car park
off Park Terrace via ramp.
Grab rails around bath only

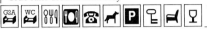

PENCOED Old Mill **MID GLAMORGAN**
Felindre Road CF3 5HU
☎ (0656) 864404 Central Res (0800) 850950
FORTE TRAVELODGE ⌂
Access through main double doors from car park
via ramp

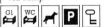

PORTHCAWL **MID GLAMORGAN**
The Promenade CF36 3LU
☎ (0656) 782261
SEABANK ⭐⭐⭐ **59%**
Access through single door via ramp

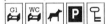

SARN PARK MOTORWAY **MID GLAMORGAN**
SERVICE AREA CF32 9RW (M4 jnct 36)
☎ Bridgend (0656) 659218 Central Res (0800) 850950
FORTE TRAVELODGE ⌂
Access through main double doors from car park
via ramp

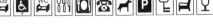

BRECON Castle Square LD3 0DB **POWYS**
☎ (0874) 624611
CASTLE OF BRECON ⭐⭐ **63%**
Access through main double doors from Castle
Square

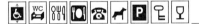

BUILTH WELLS LD2 3NP   **POWYS**
☎ (0982) 552601
CAER BERIS MANOR ★★★ **65%**
Access through main single door via ramp

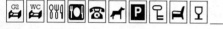

LLANGAMMARCH WELLS*   **POWYS**
LD4 4BS ☎ (05912) 202 & 474
LAKE ★★★ **76%** ⚑
Access through side single door from
Llangammarch Road

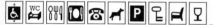

CARDIFF   **SOUTH GLAMORGAN**
Mill Lane CF1 1EZ ☎ (0222) 399944
CARDIFF MARRIOTT ★★★★ **64%**
Access through main double automatic doors
from car park off Mill Lane via ramp.
Grab rails around bath only

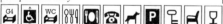

CARDIFF   **SOUTH GLAMORGAN**
Copthorne Way Culverhouse Cross CF5 6XJ
☎ (0222) 599100
COPTHORNE ★★★★ **64%**
Access through main double automatic doors off
Copthorne Way

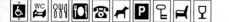

CARDIFF   **SOUTH GLAMORGAN**
Circle Way East off A48(M) Llanederyn CF3 7ND
☎ (0222) 549564 Central Res (0800) 850950
FORTE TRAVELODGE ⌂
Access through main double doors from car park
via ramp

CARDIFF   **SOUTH GLAMORGAN**
Cardiff West CF7 8SB ☎ (0222) 892255
PAVILION LODGE ⌂
Access through main double doors from car park

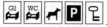

PORT TALBOT   **WEST GLAMORGAN**
SA12 6QP ☎ (0639) 884949
ABERAVAN BEACH ★★★ **58%**
Access through main double door from car park
via ramp

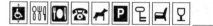

SWANSEA   **WEST GLAMORGAN**
M4 Motorway (jnct 47) ☎ (0792) 894894
PAVILION LODGE ⌂
Access through main automatic double doors
from car park

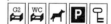

SCOTLAND

KELSO*   **BORDERS (Roxburghshire)**
36-37 The Square TD5 7HL ☎ (0573) 223303
CROSS KEYS ★★★ **58%**
Access through double swing doors from The
Square via ramp

ST BOSWELLS   **BORDERS (Roxburghshire)**
TD6 0RQ ☎ (0835) 22261
DRYBURGH ABBEY ★★★ **73%**
Access through main swing or revolving door via
ramp

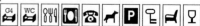

CALLANDER **CENTRAL (Perthshire)**
FK17 8BG ☎ (0877) 30003
ROMAN CAMP ★★★ **69%** 🌲

Access through main double doors

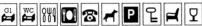

DENNY **CENTRAL (Stirlingshire)**
Fintry Road FK6 5JF ☎ (0324) 822471
THE TOPPS FH
Access through rear single door off Fintry Road via ramp. Grab rails around shower only

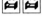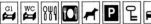

DRYMEN **CENTRAL (Stirlingshire)**
G63 0BQ ☎ (0360) 60588
BUCHANAN HIGHLAND ★★★ **65%**
Access through double doors from Main Street via ramp

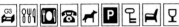

STIRLING **CENTRAL (Stirlingshire)**
Pirhall Roundabout Snabhead FK7 8EU
☎ (0786) 815033
GRANADA LODGE ⌂
Access through main swing door

DUMFRIES & GALLOWAY (Dumfriesshire)
CARRUTHERSTOWN DG1 4JX
☎ Dumfries (0387) 84201
HETLAND HALL ★★★ **65%**
Access through rear double doors

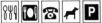

DUMFRIES & GALLOWAY (Kirkcudbrightshire)
COLVEND DG5 4QW
☎ Rockcliffe (055663) 372
CLONYARD HOUSE ★★ **67%**
Access through side double doors

DUMFRIES & GALLOWAY (Kirkcudbrightshire)
GATEHOUSE OF FLEET* DG7 2DL
☎ (0557) 814341
CALLY PALACE ★★★★ **66%**
Access through rear double doors

DUMFRIES & GALLOWAY (Dumfriesshire)
GRETNA (with Gretna Green) CA6 5HQ (on A74)
☎ (0461) 37566 Central Res (0800) 850950
FORTE TRAVELODGE ⌂
Access through main double doors from car park via ramp

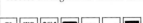

DUMFRIES & GALLOWAY (Dumfriesshire)
LOCKERBIE DG11 2SF
☎ (05762) 2427 due to change to (0576) 202427
DRYFESDALE ★★★ **66%**
Access through main double doors via ramp

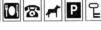

DUMFRIES & GALLOWAY (Dumfriesshire)
MOFFAT High Street DG10 9HL ☎ (0683) 20039
MOFFAT HOUSE ★★★ **65%**
Access through side double doors from High Street via ramp

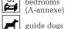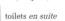

★★★★ hotel rating (see p.43)	★ Red Star highest award to hotel (see p.44)	% percentage rating (see p.44)	🌲 country house hotel (see p.44)	⌂ travel lodge (see p.43)
GH guest house	**T&C** town & country homes (see p.42)	G1 ground floor bedrooms (A-annexe)	WC toilets *en suite*	access to reception
FH farmhouse	lift	guide dogs	dining room	access to lounge
INN inn	telephone/intercom	**P** parking at entrance	room service	access to bar

* Details have not been confirmed for 1993. Please check when booking, including information about grab rails.

DUMFRIES & GALLOWAY (Dumfriesshire)
SANQUHAR Mennock DG4 6HS
☎ (0659) 50382 & 50477
MENNOCKFOOT LODGE ★★ **60%**
Access through main single door via ramp.
No grab rails in bathroom

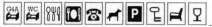

ABERDEEN **GRAMPIAN (Aberdeenshire)**
Souter Head Road Altens AB1 4LF
☎ (0224) 877000
SKEAN DHU ALTENS ★★★★ **54%**
Access through main double doors from Souter
Head Road. No grab rails in bathroom

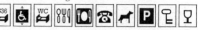

DUNFERMLINE Crossford KY12 8QW **FIFE**
☎ (0383) 736258
KEAVIL HOUSE ★★★ **66%**
Access through main single door

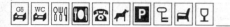

BANCHORY **GRAMPIAN (Kincardineshire)**
AB3 4ED ☎ (03302) 4884
RAEMOIR ★★★ **75%** ♨
Access through side single door via ramp

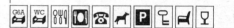

DUNFERMLINE* Aberdour Road **FIFE**
KY11 4PB ☎ (0383) 722282
PITBAUCHLIE HOUSE ★★★ **65%**
Access through double doors from Aberdour Road
via ramp

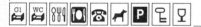

DYCE **GRAMPIAN (Aberdeenshire)**
Riverview Drive, Farburn AB2 0AZ
☎ (0224) 770011
ABERDEEN MARRIOTT ★★★★ **67%**
Access through main double doors from
Riverview Drive via one step

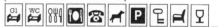

ST ANDREWS Old Station Road **FIFE**
KY16 9SP ☎ (0334) 74371
ST ANDREWS OLD COURSE
HOTEL ★★★★ Red
Access through main single door from Old Station
Road via one step

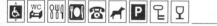

HUNTLY **GRAMPIAN (Aberdeenshire)**
AB5 4SH ☎ (0466) 792696
CASTLE ★★ **56%** ♨
Access through rear single and double doors.
Grab rails around bath only

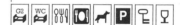

ABERDEEN* **GRAMPIAN (Aberdeenshire)**
122 Huntly Street AB1 1SU
☎ (0224) 630404
COPTHORNE ★★★ **67%**
Access through car park lift from Huntly Street

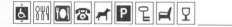

AVIEMORE **HIGHLAND (Inverness-shire)**
Aviemore Centre PH22 1PF ☎ (0479) 810681
STAKIS AVIEMORE
FOUR SEASONS ★★★★ **58%**
Access through main automatic door from
Aviemore Centre

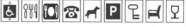

ABERDEEN **GRAMPIAN (Aberdeenshire)**
Waterton Road AB2 9HS ☎ (0224) 712275
THE CRAIGHAR ★★★ **66%**
Access through main double doors from car park
off Waterton Road via one step

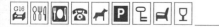

BRORA* **HIGHLAND (Sutherland)**
Golf Road KW9 6QS ☎ (0408) 621225
THE LINKS ★★★ **56%**
Access through main double swing doors from
Golf Road via ramp

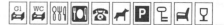

CONTIN IV14 9EY **HIGHLAND (Ross-shire)**
☎ Strathpeffer (0997) 421487
COUL HOUSE ★★★ 68% ♨♣
Access through main single door from car park via ramp

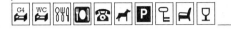

MEY KW14 8XH **HIGHLAND (Caithness)**
☎ Barrock (084785) 244
CASTLE ARMS ★★ 59%
Access through side/rear single door from car park via ramp

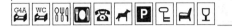

DALWHINNIE* **HIGHLAND (Inverness-shire)**
PA19 1AF ☎ (05282) 257
LOCH ERICHT ★★ 59%
Access through main single swing door from Main Road via ramp

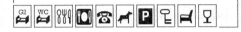

ONICH **HIGHLAND (Inverness-shire)**
Creag Dhu PH33 6RY ☎ (08553) 237
LODGE ON THE LOCH ★★★ 65%
Access through side single swing door from car park

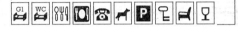

INVERNESS **HIGHLAND (Inverness-shire)**
11 Culduthel Road IV2 4AG ☎ (0463) 222897
BEAUFORT ★★ 60%
Access through rear swing door from Culduthel Road via ramp

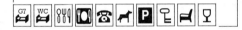

SPEAN BRIDGE **HIGHLAND (Inverness-shire)**
PH34 4ES ☎ (039781) 250
SPEAN BRIDGE ★★ 59%
Access through main single and double doors from car park

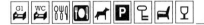

INVERNESS **HIGHLAND (Inverness-shire)**
10 Ness Bank IV2 4SG ☎ (0463) 234308
GLEN MHOR ★★ 69%
Access through single swing door from car park off Ness Bank via ramp

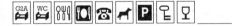

ABERLADY* **LOTHIAN (East Lothian)**
Main Street EH32 0RE ☎ (08757) 682
KILSPINDIE HOUSE ★★ 66%
Access through main single door via one step

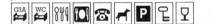

INVERNESS **HIGHLAND (Inverness-shire)**
Culcabock Road IV2 3LP ☎ (0463) 237166
KINGSMILLS HOTEL ★★★★ 66%
Access through main automatic doors from Culcabock Road

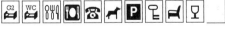

EDINBURGH **LOTHIAN (Midlothian)**
Princes Street EH1 2AB ☎ 031-225 2433
CALEDONIAN ★★★★★ 69%
Access through main swing and revolving doors from Princes Street via two steps

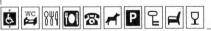

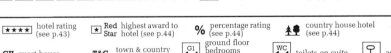

★★★★ hotel rating (see p.43)	★ Red highest award to Star hotel (see p.44)	% percentage rating (see p.44)	♨♣ country house hotel (see p.44) ⌂ travel lodge (see p.43)
GH guest house	T&C town & country homes (see p.42)	G1 ground floor bedrooms (A-annexe)	WC toilets *en suite* ♿ access to reception
FH farmhouse	🔲 lift	guide dogs	dining room access to lounge
INN inn	☎ telephone/intercom	P parking at entrance	room service access to bar
* Details have not been confirmed for 1993. Please check when booking, including information about grab rails.			

EDINBURGH **LOTHIAN (Midlothian)**
Clermiston Road EH12 6UG ☎ 031-334 3391
CAPITAL MOAT HOUSE ★★★ 65%
Access through main double swing doors from car park off Clermiston Road via ramp

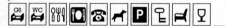

EDINBURGH **LOTHIAN (Midlothian)**
North Bridge EH1 1SD ☎ 031-556 7277
CARLTON HIGHLAND ★★★★ 68%
Access through main single and revolving doors from North Bridge

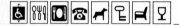

EDINBURGH* **LOTHIAN (Midlothian)**
4 Ellersley Road ☎ 031-337 6888
ELLERSLEY HOUSE ★★★ 54%
Access through double doors from Ellersley Road via ramp

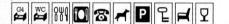

EDINBURGH **LOTHIAN (Midlothian)**
Dreghorn Link ☎ 031-441 4296
Central Res (0800) 850950
FORTE TRAVELODGE ⌂
Access through main double doors from car park via ramp

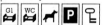

EDINBURGH* **LOTHIAN (Midlothian)**
Grosvenor Street ☎ 031-226 6001
STAKIS EDINBURGH GROSVENOR ★★★ 63%
Access through side double doors from Grosvenor Street via ramp

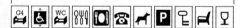

MUSSELBURGH **LOTHIAN (Midlothian)**
A1 Old Craighall EH21 8RE ☎ 031-653 2427
GRANADA LODGE ⌂
Access through double doors from car park

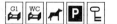

STRATHCLYDE (Dunbartonshire)
DUMBARTON Milton G82 2TY
☎ (0389) 65202 Central Res (0800) 850950
FORTE TRAVELODGE ⌂
Access through main double doors from car park via ramp

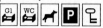

CONNEL **STRATHCLYDE (Argyllshire)**
PA37 1PB ☎ (063171) 483
FALLS OF LORA ★★ 65%
Access through rear single door via ramp

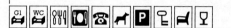

ERISKA **STRATHCLYDE (Argyllshire)**
PA37 1SD ☎ Ledaig (063172) 371
ISLE OF ERISKA ★★★ Red ⚜
Access through double doors from car park via ramp

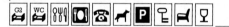

ERSKINE* **STRATHCLYDE (Renfrewshire)**
North Barr PA8 6AN ☎ 041-812 0123
FORTE POSTHOUSE GLASGOW ★★★ 67%
Access through main double swing doors via one step

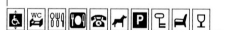

GLASGOW* **STRATHCLYDE (Lanarkshire)**
99 Gordon Street G1 3SF ☎ 041-221 9680
CENTRAL ★★★ 59%
Access through rear double doors from BR Station or concourse

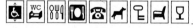

GLASGOW **STRATHCLYDE (Lanarkshire)**
Argyle Street Anderston G3 8RR ☎ 041-226 5577
GLASGOW MARRIOTT ★★★★ 62%
Access through main automatic doors from Argyle Street

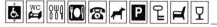

GLASGOW	STRATHCLYDE (Lanarkshire)

Great Western Road G12 0XP ☎ 041-334 8161
JURYS POND ★★★ **60%**
Access through main double doors from Great
Western Road via ramp. No grab rails in
bathroom

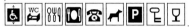

GLASGOW	STRATHCLYDE (Lanarkshire)

Congress Road G3 8QT ☎ 041-204 0733
MOAT HOUSE INTERNATIONAL ★★★★ **69%**
Access through main double swing and revolving
doors from Congress Road

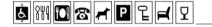

GLASGOW	STRATHCLYDE (Lanarkshire)

1/10 Grosvenor Terrace G12 0TA ☎ 041-339 8811
STAKIS GROSVENOR ★★★★ **60%**
Access through double revolving doors from
Grosvenor Terrace via ramp.
No grab rails in bathroom

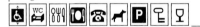

LARGS	STRATHCLYDE (Ayrshire)

Greenock Road KA30 8QL ☎ (0475) 673119
SPRINGFIELD ★★ **59%**
Access through main swing doors from Greenock
Road via ramp

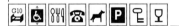

OBAN*	STRATHCLYDE (Argyllshire)

Corran Esplanade PA34 5AA ☎ (0631) 62381
ALEXANDRA ★★★ **60%**
Access through single door from Esplanade via
ramp

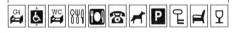

RHU*	STRATHCLYDE (Dunbartonshire)

G84 8NF ☎ (0436) 820684
ROSSLEA HALL ★★★
Access through main double swing doors from
Ferry Road via ramp

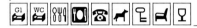

STRACHUR*	STRATHCLYDE (Argyllshire)

PA27 8BX ☎ (036986) 279
CREGGANS INN ★★★ **65%**
Access through main and rear single doors via
ramp

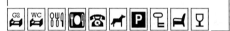

TROON	STRATHCLYDE (Ayrshire)

KA10 6HE ☎ (0292) 314444
MARINE HIGHLAND ★★★★ **65%**
Access through double swing doors from Crosbie
Road via ramp

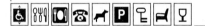

TURNBERRY	STRATHCLYDE (Ayrshire)

KA26 9LT ☎ (0655) 31000
TURNBERRY HOTEL ★★★★★ **73%**
Access through main revolving and single door
via one step. No grab rails in bathroom

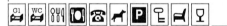

UDDINGSTON*	STRATHCLYDE (Lanarkshire)

8-10 Glasgow Road G71 7AS
☎ (0698) 813774 & 814843
REDSTONES ★★ **64%**
Access through double doors from car park off
Brooklands Avenue

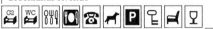

AUCHTERARDER | **TAYSIDE (Perthshire)**

PH3 1NF ☎ (0764) 62231
GLENEAGLES ★★★★★ Red
Access through double doors via ramp

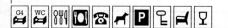

BLAIRGOWRIE | **TAYSIDE (Perthshire)**

PH10 6SG ☎ (0250) 884237
KINLOCH HOUSE ★★★ 77%
Access through main single doors via ramp

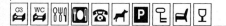

DUNDEE* | **TAYSIDE (Angus)**

Kingsway West Invergowrie DD2 5JT
☎ (0382) 641122
SWALLOW ★★★ 65%
Access through double doors from car park

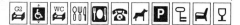

DUNKELD | **TAYSIDE (Perthshire)**

Birnam PH8 0BQ ☎ (0350) 727462
BIRNAM ★★★ 63%
*Access through main double doors from Perth
Road. No grab rails in bathroom*

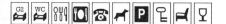

KINCLAVEN* | **TAYSIDE (Perthshire)**

PH1 4QN ☎ Meikleour (0250) 883268
BALLATHIE HOUSE ★★★ 77% ♠
*Access through main door via one step or side
door via ramp*

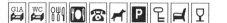

KINNESSWOOD | **TAYSIDE (Kinross-shire)**

KY13 7HN ☎ (0592) 84253
LOMOND COUNTRY INN ★★ 65%
*Access through single door from car park via one
step*

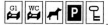

KINROSS | **TAYSIDE (Kinross-shire)**

Kincardine Road KY13 7NQ ☎ (0577) 64646
GRANADA LODGE ⌂
Access through main double doors via ramp

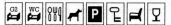

KIRKMICHAEL | **TAYSIDE (Perthshire)**

PH10 7NB ☎ Strathardle (0250) 881288
LOG CABIN ★★ 61%
Access through side single door via ramp

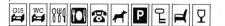

MONTROSE | **TAYSIDE (Angus)**

61 John Street DD10 8RJ ☎ (0674) 73415
PARK ★★★ 59%
*Access through single door from car park via one
step. Grab rails around bath only*

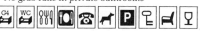

PERTH | **TAYSIDE (Perthshire)**

St Leonards Bank PH2 8EB ☎ (0738) 22451
PARKLANDS ★★★ 73%
*Access through single door from car park off
Marshall Place via two steps.
No grab rails in private bathrooms*

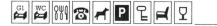

PITLOCHRY* | **TAYSIDE (Perthshire)**

West Moulin Road PH16 5EQ ☎ (0796) 472399
CRAIGVRACK ★★ 62%
*Access through main double doors from West
Moulin Road via ramp*

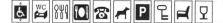

PITLOCHRY | **TAYSIDE (Perthshire)**

Knockard Road PH16 5JH ☎ (0796) 472666
PITLOCHRY HYDRO ★★★ 65%
*Access through main sliding door from Knockard
Road via ramp. No grab rails in bathrooms*

IRELAND

ENNIS Clare Road **CO CLARE**
☎ (065) 28421
WEST COUNTRY INN ★★★ **58%**
Access through double swing doors via one step

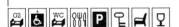

NEWMARKET-ON-FERGUS **CO CLARE**
☎ (061) 368161
CLARE INN ★★★ **63%**
Access through main double and single doors via ramp. Grab rails around bath only

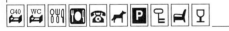

SHANNON Shannon Airport **CO CLARE**
☎ (061) 471122
THE GREAT SOUTHERN ★★★★ **59%**
Access through main double swing doors from Airport Road via ramp

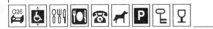

BLARNEY ☎ (021) 385281 **CO CORK**
BLARNEY PARK ★★★ **68%**
Access through main single door via ramp

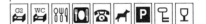

CORK Western Road **CO CORK**
☎ (021) 276622
JURYS HOTEL ★★★★ **66%**
Access through main double doors from Western Road

KINSALE Worlds End **CO CORK**
☎ (021) 772301
TRIDENT ★★★ **70%**
Access through main double doors from car park off Pier Road via ramp. No grab rails in bathroom

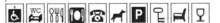

★★★★	hotel rating (see p.43)	★	Red Star	highest award to hotel (see p.44)	%	percentage rating (see p.44)	▲♣	country house hotel (see p.44)	⌂	travel lodge (see p.43)
GH	guest house	**T&C**		town & country homes (see p.42)	G1	ground floor bedrooms (A-annexe)	WC		toilets *en suite*		access to reception
FH	farmhouse			lift			guide dogs			dining room		access to lounge
INN	inn			telephone/ intercom	**P**	parking at entrance			room service		access to bar

* Details have not been confirmed for 1993. Please check when booking, including information about grab rails.

HOLYWOOD BT18 0EX CO DOWN
☎ (0232) 425223
CULLODEN ★★★★ **70%**
Access through main automatic double doors from Bangor Road via ramp

---

DUBLIN Ballsbridge CO DUBLIN
☎ (01) 605000
JURYS ★★★★ **64%**
Access through main swing and revolving doors from Pembroke Road

---

DUN LAOGHAIRE CO DUBLIN
Rochestown Avenue ☎ (01) 2853555
VICTOR ★★★ **59%**
Access through main single door from Rochestown Avenue via ramp

---

LUCAN CO DUBLIN
☎ (01) 6280494
LUCAN SPA ★★★ **54%**
Access through main single door via ramp

KILLARNEY CO KERRY
☎ (064) 31144
CASTLEROSSE ★★★ **64%**
Access through main double doors

KILLARNEY Muckross Road CO KERRY
☎ (064) 31035
LAKE ★★★ **57%**
Access through main double doors from Muckross Road. Grab rails around bath only

---

TRALEE Killarney Road CO KERRY
☎ (066) 21299
EARL OF DESMOND ★★★ **58%**
Access through main double doors via ramp

KILKENNY College Road CO KILKENNY
☎ (056) 62000
KILKENNY ★★★ **65%**
Access through side double doors from College Road. No grab rails in bathroom

---

KILKENNY CO KILKENNY
☎ (056) 22122
NEWPARK HOTEL ★★★ **65%**
Access through main single and double sliding doors from Castlecombe Road

---

WESTPORT CO MAYO
☎ (098) 25122
HOTEL WESTPORT ★★★ **61%**
Access through side double door via ramp

ATHLONE Mardyke Street CO WESTMEATH
☎ (0902) 72924
ROYAL HOEY ★★ **68%**
Access through main double doors from Mardyke Street via one step. Grab rails around bath only

---

ROSSLARE CO WEXFORD
☎ (053) 32114
KELLY'S ★★★ Red
Access through main swing door via ramp

HOTELS SUITABLE FOR DINING ONLY

The following hotels are not suitable for accommodation purposes, however, their restaurants are suitable. We advise you to check when booking to ensure the facilities are suited to your particular disability. Where a tick is shown in the 'Public toilet adjoining restaurant' column, the establishment concerned has indicated that these facilities are suitable for disabled people.

au	automatic doors	cp	car park	d	double doors
md	main door	n	normal doors	r	ramp
sd	side door	sl	sliding doors	sw	swing
re	rear	el	electric		

Country/ County/Town	Classification	Establishment Address	Telephone Number	Entrance	No. of steps to entrance	Type of door at entrance	No. of steps to restaurant	Public toilet adj. restaurant
ENGLAND								
Cambridgeshire								
Bar Hill	★★★	Cambridgeshire Moat House	Crafts Hill (0954) 780555	md	–	av/ sl	–	–
St Ives	★★★	Olivers Lodge Needingworth Road	Huntingdon (0480) 63252	re	1	d	–	√
Cheshire								
Alderley Edge	★★★	Alderley Edge Macclesfield Road	(0625) 583033	md	r	d	–	√
Sandbach	★★★	Saxon Cross Holmes Chapel Road	Crewe (0270) 763281	md	–	d/ sw	–	√
Cleveland								
Stockton-on-Tees	★★★★	Swallow 10 John Walker Square	(0642) 679721	md	1	–	–	–
Cornwall								
Newquay	★★	Tremont Pentire Avenue	(0637) 872984	md	–	d	–	√
St Agnes	★	Sunholme Goonvrea Road	(0872) 552318	md	2	n	–	–
Cumbria								
Grasmere	★★★★	Wordsworth	(05394) 35592	md	1	n	–	√

Country/ County/Town	Classification	Establishment Address	Telephone Number	Entrance	No. of steps to entrance	Type of door at entrance	No. of steps to restaurant	Public toilet adj. restaurant
Devon								
Barnstaple	★★★	Barnstaple Motel Braunton Road	(0271) 76221	sd	r	d	–	–
Exeter	★★★	Countess Wear Lodge Topsham Road	Topsham (0392) 875441	md	r	d	–	√
Torquay	★★	Seascape 8-10 Tor Church Road	(0803) 292617	md	2	d/ sw	–	–
East Sussex								
Halland	★★	Halland Forge	(0825) 840456	md	–	d	–	√
Gloucestershire								
Lower Slaughter	★★★	Washbourne Court	(0451) 822143	md	–	n	–	–
Tetbury	★★★	Hare & Hounds Westonbirt	(0666) 880233	md	r	d	–	–
Hampshire								
Basingstoke	★★★	Centrecourt Centre Drive Chineham	(0256) 816664	md	–	d/ sw	–	√
Rotherwick	★★★★ ♨	Tylney Hall	(0256) 764881	md	–	d	–	√
Hereford & Worcester								
Evesham	★★★	Evesham Coopers Lane off Waterside	(0386) 765566	md	–	n	–	
Ross-on-Wye	★★ ♨	Peterstow Country House Peterstow	(0989) 62826	md	–	n	–	√
Hertfordshire								
Harpenden	★★★	Harpenden Moat House 18 Southdown Road	(0582) 764111	md	1	d	–	–
Watford	★★★	Dean Park 30-40 St Albans Road	(0923) 229212	md	r	d	–	–
Kent								
Ashford	★★★	Master Spearpoint Canterbury Road Kennington	(0233) 636863	md	r	n	–	–
Sevenoaks	★★★	Royal Oak Upper High Street	(0732) 451109	md	1	sw	–	–
Lancashire								
Bury	★★★	Normandie Elbut Lane Birtle	061-764 3869	md	r	d	–	–
London (Central)								
W1	★★★★★	Mayfair Inter-Continental Stratton Street	071-629 7777	md	r	sw	–	√
W2	★★★★	Royal Lancaster Lancaster Terrace	071-262 6737	md	r	d/ sw	–	√

Country/ County/Town	Classification	Establishment Address	Telephone Number	Entrance	No. of steps to entrance	Type of door at entrance	No. of steps to restaurant	Public toilet adj. restaurant
Northamptonshire Wellingborough	★★★	Hind, Sheep Street	(0933) 22287	md	r	d	–	√
North Yorkshire Easingwold	★★	George Market Place	(0347) 21698	re	r	n	1	–
Settle	★★★	Falcon Manor Skipton Road	(0729) 823814	md	1	n	–	–
York	★★★★	Viking North Street	(0904) 659822	cp	–	–	–	–
Oxfordshire Burford	★★	Cotswold Gateway Cheltenham Road	(099382) 2695	md	r	d/ sw	–	√
South Yorkshire Doncaster	★★★	Danum Swallow High Street	(0302) 342261	re	r	–	–	√
Sheffield	★★★	Charnwood 10 Sharrow Lane	(0742) 589411	cp	r	n & d	–	√
	★★★	Swallow Kenwood Road	(0742) 583811	md	r	d/ sw	–	–
Staffordshire Rugeley	★★	Cedar Tree Main Road Brereton	(0889) 584241	md	2	d	–	√
Warwickshire Stratford-upon-Avon	★★★	Falcon, Chapel Street	(0789) 205777	re	r	d	–	–
West Midlands Walsall	★★★	Beverley 58 Lichfield Road	(0922) 614967	md	1	sw	–	–
Wolverhampton	★★	Ely House 53 Tettenhall Road	(0902) 311311	re	1	n & d	–	–
West Sussex Copthorne	★★★★	Copthorne Copthorne Road	(0342) 714971	md	r	d/ sw	–	–
Crawley	★★★	Gatwick Concorde Church Road Lowfield Heath	(0293) 533441	md	–	d	–	–
West Chiltington	★★★	Roundabout Monkmead Lane	(0798) 813838	md	r	n	–	–
West Yorkshire Leeds	★★★	Stakis Windmill	(0532) 732323	md	1	sw	–	–

Country/ County/Town	Classification	Establishment Address	Telephone Number	Entrance	No. of steps to entrance	Type of door at entrance	No. of steps to restaurant	Public toilet adj. restaurant
CHANNEL ISLANDS								
Jersey Gorey	★★★	Old Court House	(0534) 54444	md	–	d	–	–
WALES								
Clwyd Northup Hall	★★★	Chequers Country House	Deeside (0244) 816181	sd	–	n	1	√
Gwent Newport	★★★	Newport Lodge Bryn Bevan	(0633) 821818	md	r	d	–	√
Gwynedd Criccieth	★★★ ♨	Bron Eifion Country House	(0766) 522385	md	1	n	–	√
Holyhead	★★	Bull London Road Valley	(0407) 740351	re	–	n	–	√
SCOTLAND								
Borders Galashiels (Selkirkshire)	★★	Abbotsford Arms 63 Stirling Street	(0896) 2517	md	1	n	–	√
Dumfries & Galloway Newton Stewart (Wigtownshire)	★★	Creebridge House	(0671) 2121	re	r	n	1	√
Grampian Inverurie (Aberdeenshire)	★★★	Strathburn Burghmuir Drive	(0467) 24422	md	r	n	–	√
Highland Contin (Ross-shire)	★★	Craigdarroch Lodge Craigdarroch Drive	Strathpeffer (0997) 421265	md	–	d	–	–
Fort William (Inverness-shire)	★★★	Moorings Banavie	Corpach (0397) 772797	md	1	d	–	√
Kyle of Lochalsh (Ross-shire)	★★	Kyle Main Street	(0599) 4204	sd	r	d	–	–
Lairg (Sutherland)	★★★	Sutherland Arms	(0549) 2291	md	–	d	–	–

Country/ County/Town	Classification	Establishment Address	Telephone Number	Entrance	No. of steps to entrance	Type of door at entrance	No. of steps to restaurant	Public toilet adj. restaurant
Strathclyde Renfrew	★★★	Dean Park 91 Glasgow Road	041-886 3771	md	r	–	1	√
Tayside Pitlochry	★★	Castlebeigh House 10 Knockard Road	(0796) 472925	md	2	n	–	√
Shetland Lerwick	★★★	Lerwick South Road	(0595) 2166	md	–	d	–	√
IRELAND								
Co Donegal Dunfanaghy	★★	Carrig Rua	(074) 36133	md	r	n	–	√

SPECIALISED ACCOMMODATION

There are a number of organisations which offer specialised holiday accommodation for the disabled which is up to hotel standards:

John Grooms Association for the Disabled
Has two award-winning hotels providing seaside accommodation for those in wheelchairs, the Promenade at Minehead (Somerset) and the West Shore at Llandudno (Gwynedd) – further details under placename in directory
    Set in the Vale of Glamorgan near Cowbridge, the Association's newest hotel, the Jane Hodge Hotel and Activities Centre is a purpose-designed and built hotel and activities centre for disabled people, their family, friends and escorts. The hotel has 30 twin-bedded rooms situated on the ground floor with en suite facilities and with easy electric door unlock system. There are adjoining family rooms and a care room, one specially for blind people and one for deaf people. Facilities for leisure activities include snooker, table tennis, wheelchair hockey and dancing, a swimming pool, jacuzzi and sauna.

The Association also provides self-catering accommodation (see under heading Self-Catering for further details). Guests are asked to bring able-bodied friends to provide any help needed. The Association has also taken over the Visitors Club, which offers reduced rates at the London Tara Hotel. Membership of the club is £3 (£5 overseas membership). For full details of all the above schemes contact: Holidays Administrator, John Grooms Association for the Disabled, 10 Gloucester Drive, Finsbury Park, London N4 2LP tel 081-800 8695/6.

> **Although the accommodation has not been inspected by the AA to date the following organisations are among those who also offer this type of holiday.**

Trefoil Holiday Centre for the Disabled
Specially designed holiday accommodation catering for individuals and groups of up to 40 handicapped people of all ages. Features

include an indoor heated swimming pool, games room, softplay room, bar, shop and an 16-seater bus equipped with lift. Guests who need help must bring an able-bodied escort. Bookings to: The Warden, Miss G. Macpherson, The Trefoil Centre, Gogarbank, Edinburgh EH12 9DA *tel* 031-339 3148.

The Winged Fellowship

Specialises in providing holidays and respite care for physically disabled people. It has five Holiday Centres in Surrey, Essex, Nottingham, Southampton and Southport. Regular entertainment and outings are provided in an informal atmosphere. Most Centres have a swimming pool and craft room. Volunteers work alongside fully qualified staff to ensure maximum comfort and variety of opportunity for the guests. Special activity weeks are arranged including music, drama, youth fortnights, etc. Open February-December. Minimum

age 16. UK touring holidays and holidays abroad are also arranged. (See section: The Disabled Traveller Abroad page 135 for further details). Full colour brochure from: Winged Fellowship Trust, Angel House, 20/32 Pentonville Road, London N1 9XD *tel* 071-833 2594.

Kiltrasna Farm

Muckross, Killarney, Co. Kerry, Eire (Mrs C. Looney *tel* 010-353-64 31643). Accommodation in a comfortable ranch-type bungalow guesthouse on a working farm. B&B or full-board. Details from Mrs E. Ashton Edwards *tel* 081-940 2276.

Bryn Meirion Guest House

Tim and Chris Holland, Bryn Meirion Guest House, Amlwch Road, Benllech, Anglesey LL74 8SR *tel* (0248) 853118. A family run guest house, adapted with the wheelchair user in mind, set in lawned gardens on the eastern coast of the island. Special diets can be catered for.

SELF-CATERING

The following organisations offer AA recommended holiday cottages adapted to suit the needs of disabled people:

Clwyd

The Firs, Mold, Clwyd. Modern bungalow specially adapted and furnished for the needs of the wheelchair-bound visitor. Comprise lounge/diner, kitchen, utility room, bathroom/WC (with additional disabled person's bathroom), two bedrooms and a sun lounge. Private rear garden and telephone. Sleeps four. For bookings: Lynne James, 7 Overpool Road, Ellesmere Port, South Wirral L66 4NF *tel* 051-339 5316.

Cornwall

R. R. & N. G. Hall, Penrose Burden, St Breward, Bodmin, Cornwall PL30 4LZ *tel* Bodmin (0208) 850277 and 850617. Eight traditional stone cottages sleeping 2–6 (two, riverside with fishing). Each has excellent access (off tarmac) and amenities designed by the owner, who is himself disabled, to suit wheelchair users. Car essential. Meals on arrival and evening meals available if required. Highly Commended (1992) by the Holiday Care Service (see page 124).

Janet and Christopher Ridley, Trenillocs, St Columb Major, Cornwall TR9 6JN *tel* (0637) 880394. 'Bowjyrooz' is a luxury conversion of a stone and slate barn, done with the wheelchair-disabled in mind. Situated on a small farm in a peaceful area of North Cornwall, the view across the valley and private trout stream is most restful. The ground floor includes a lounge/diner with open fireplace, kitchen, shower/laundry-room with WC, and a games-room with table-tennis and darts. Upstairs (Stannah stairlift) there are three bedrooms, double, twin and single, and bathroom with WC and bidet. Central heating throughout. Leaflet gives details.

Cumbria

Beck Allans Holiday Apartments, College Street, Grasmere, Cumbria. A ground floor apartment offering very comfortable accommodation but having no special facilities for the disabled and therefore perhaps more suitable for those clients with some mobility. Lies in centre of the village in own well timbered grounds, car parking etc. For full details: Mrs Pat Taylor, Beck Allans,

College Street, Grasmere, Cumbria LA22 9SZ *tel* (05394) 35563.

'Deloraine', a spacious Edwardian mansion, situated in a secluded, elevated position near Lake Windermere offers comfortable accommodation for the disabled in the ground floor flat – 'Brant'. In addition the larger 'Birch Cottage' adjoining, a converted stone and slate building in the grounds, offers 'home-comfort' accommodation for disabled and able-bodied alike. Both have easy level access, parking adjoining and bathroom adaptations. For full details: Mrs P. M. Fanstone, Deloraine, Helm Road, Windermere, Cumbria LA23 2HS *tel* Windermere (05394) 45557.

Dyfed

Mr J. E. Lloyd, Rosemoor, Walwyn's Castle, Haverfordwest, Dyfed *tel* Broadhaven (0437) 781326. Four cottages suitable for the disabled person who is accompanied by an able-bodied person. One unit has a bedroom with en suite bathroom which has been designed with professional advice. Situated within the Rosemoor Estate, a nature reserve for migratory and breeding birds.

Gwynedd

Menai Holidays, Capel Ogwen, Penrhyn Park, Bangor, Gwynedd. Large house in walled garden on coastline. The ground floor includes a lounge/diner, kitchen, games room, WC and twin-bedded room, suitable for disabled. The house has five further bedrooms with two bathrooms. Also two converted farmhouses, Moelfre and Brynsiencyn, at Anglesey, close to the sea. Both have a shower room and WC en suite in a downstairs bedroom and ramps for wheelchairs. Enquiries to: Menai Holidays, The Old Port Office, Port Penrhyn, Bangor, Gwynedd LL57 4HN *tel* Bangor (0248) 351055.

Inverness-shire

David Turner, Dunsmore Lodges, Farley, Beauly, Inverness-shire IV4 7EY *tel* Beauly (0463) 782424. Very comfortable Scandinavian-style chalet specially designed for disabled guests, set in beautiful Highlands of Scotland. Open mid March to October. Free colour brochure available.

Although the following accommodation has not necessarily been inspected by the AA to date the following organisations/ individuals are among those who offer this type of holiday.

John Grooms Association

John Grooms Association for the Disabled. Three bungalows, two chalets and one London flat, adapted to suit disabled visitors, at a choice of five locations. Also mobile holiday homes at a choice of seven locations. Each mobile home is specially designed for wheelchair use with ramped entrance, wide doors and corridors, low windows, wheelchair-toilet and shower. For bookings see entry for John Grooms, under Specialised Accommodation, page 103.

Youth Hostels Association

The YHA welcomes hostellers, individuals or small groups of people who need a wheelchair to get around or who have visual, hearing or other handicaps. We have many positive advantages to offer, above all friendly companionship and inexpensive accommodation. Although some of our Youth Hostels are designed to cater for people with disabilities, (Broadhaven and Manorbier for example), other Hostels do vary in terms of accessibility particularly for wheelchairs. In view of this we recommend that you telephone or visit (especially if you are intending to take a group) the Hostel in advance to discuss your requirements and the facilities available at the Hostel. The warden will be more than pleased to help you. For further details please contact: Youth Hostels Association, Trevelyan House, 8 St Stephens Hill, St Albans, Herts AL1 2DY *tel* (0727) 55215.

Aberdeenshire

Gordon Holiday Cottages, Gartly, near Huntly, Aberdeenshire. Modernised cottage but retaining its original character, providing accommodation for the seriously disabled complying to the standards of the Scottish Tourist Board for wheelchair visitors. Accommodation comprises lounge/bedroom/kitchen, bathroom/WC, and a double bedroom. Situated in village centre. An adjoining two-bedroomed cottage for larger groups is available and is suitable for the more mobile disabled. For bookings: Mr J. T. Cosgrove,

118 Kidmore End Road, Emmer Green, Reading RG4 8SL *tel* Reading (0734) 472524.

Cumbria

Mr Massingham, Crossfield Farm, Kirkoswald, Penrith, Cumbria CA10 1EU *tel* (0768) 898711. Cottage complex situated in secluded rural location. Level access throughout. Assistance for wheelchair user to adjacent fishing area.

Mr & Mrs M. R. Shallcross, The Moss, Newbiggin-on-Lune, Kirkby Stephen, Cumbria CA17 4NB *tel* Newbiggin-on-Lune (05396) 23316. Two cottages specially converted to suit disabled persons, having ramped entrances, extra wide doors and appropriate bathroom facilities. Evening meal available on night of arrival. Short winter breaks (November-March) a speciality, please send for brochure.

Derbyshire

Sue and Terry Prince, The Cottage By The Pond, Beechenhill Farm, Ilam, Ashbourne, Derbyshire DE6 2BD *tel* Alstonefield (033527) 274. This beautifully decorated and furnished converted barn looks south over the counties of Derbyshire, Staffordshire and distant Leicestershire. The warm cottage is very well equipped and has been carefully designed to provide everybody (particularly those with special needs or wheelchairs) with a wonderful holiday base.

Dyfed

Patrick and Catherine McLoughlin opened Llety Mieri holiday cottages in March 1992. Three cottages, converted from stone farm buildings, offer level access, grab rails, doors wide enough for wheelchairs and over-bed hoists. Each cottage has central heating, electric cooker, colour TV and a separate laundry room. The three acres of ground are level and wild deer, herons and kingfishers can often be seen. For further details and brochure contact: Catherine McLoughlin, Hamdden Llety Meiri, Golden Grove, Carmarthen, Dyfed SA32 8NL *tel* Llandeilo (0558) 823059.

Gloucestershire

Mrs D. J. Charlton, Tibblestone Farm, Teddington, Near Tewkesbury, Gloucestershire GL20 8JA *tel* (0242) 620298. Working cattle farm with twin-bedded room on ground floor suitable for a wheelchair. Large double doors into TV lounge and dining room. Ramp access through front door. Enquiries welcome before 9.30am and after 4pm.

Kent

Mr & Mrs Topping, Misling Farm, Stelling Minnis, Stone Street, Canterbury, Kent CT4 6DE *tel* Stelling Minnis (022787) 256. A carefully-converted 18th-century dairy cottage providing accommodation for one accompanied disabled person with their family.

Suffolk

Mr and Mrs G. Clarke, Monk Soham Hall, Monk Soham, Woodbridge, Suffolk IP13 7EN *tel* (0728) 685358. Originally a farm building, St Peter's View has been converted to provide four properties which cater for the needs of wheelchair users. One property offers one double bedded and one twin-bedded bedroom, bath with private facilities and the three others have either one double bedded *or* one twin bedded bedroom with en suite facilities. Outside, there is a parking area adjacent to the properties and a level patio with garden furniture. All external entrances are ramped where necessary. Send for brochure.

Worcestershire

Mr & Mrs D. Berisford, Whitewells Farm, Ridgway Cross, Malvern, Worcestershire WR13 5JS *tel* Ridgway Cross (0886) 880607. A converted Tudor-style farm cottage designed for the disabled, level access.

Wight, Isle of

The Old Club House of the Royal Isle of Wight Golf Links is an all-wood building that has been converted for use as a holiday home. Situated 100 yards from the seashore and $1/4$ mile from the village of St Helen's, it is in a superb location for holidays for the accompanied disabled. Accommodation comprises two twin bedrooms with en suite facilities and one single bedroom. One of the twin bedrooms and bathroom is suitable for the disabled. For full details: The National Trust, 35a St James's Street, Newport, Isle of Wight *tel* (0983) 526445.

RECREATIONAL CENTRES

Blencathra Centre

Blencathra Centre, Threlkeld, Keswick, Cumbria CA12 4SG *tel* Threlkeld (07687) 79601. The centre is situated 1,000ft up on the slopes of Blencathra with panoramic views over the surrounding Lakeland fells. On the western aspect of the spacious grounds, four cottages have been modernised for family accommodation, whilst at the other end of the 11 acre site the main buildings have been converted into compact, self-contained hostels for group use. Some of the cottages and hostels have been adapted to cater for the disabled. For further information please send a SAE to the Manager.

Gorslwyd Farm

Gorslwyd Farm is a holiday and recreational centre which makes the countryside accessible to disabled people. Gorslwyd offers self-catering family accommodation in eight country-style cottages sleeping 6–8 persons and is accessible to a wheelchair user throughout. Designed to be enjoyed by disabled and able-bodied people: facilities include a games room, craft workshop, gardens, nature trail and adventure playground. Send a SAE for details to Bob and Jennie Donaldson, Gorslwyd Farm, Tan-y-Groes, Cardigan, Dyfed SA43 2HZ *tel* Cardigan (0239) 810593.

The Stackpole Centre

The Stackpole Centre is a holiday and study facility designed and equipped for people who have any form of disability. It is intended for use by individuals, groups or families who wish to take advantage of opportunities not normally available to them. The centre is comprised of seven self-catering cottages, two group houses, an indoor swimming pool, a small shop, a launderette and a large room for recreation or meetings. Visitors to the centre can participate in the many activities including canoeing, abseiling, horse-riding, fishing, walking, sand-yachting, birdwatching and sketching. Full details from: The Administrator, The Stackpole Centre, Home Farm, Stackpole, Pembroke, Dyfed SA71 5DQ *tel* (0646) 661425 *fax* (0646) 661456.

The Calvert Trust Kielder

The Calvert Trust Kielder, situated in the beautiful North Tyne Valley, was purpose built to offer holidays to disabled people, their family and friends. A wide range of sporting activities are offered, these include sailing, canoeing, climbing, horse riding in the forest or indoor school, archery, orienteering, target shooting, fishing and bird watching. Friendly experienced staff are on hand to give tuition, and all equipment is supplied. Fully licensed, there is also an indoor heated pool, staffed renal dialysis unit and 3 self catering chalets. Whether holidaying alone or with the family, a warm welcome awaits you at the Calvert Trust Kielder. Open all year. Highly Commended (1992) by the Holiday Care Service (see page 124). Full details from: The Director, Calvert Trust Kielder, Kielder Water, Hexham, Northumberland NE48 1BS *tel* (0434) 250232.

MOTORWAY SERVICE AREAS

Hitherto, the Automobile Association has conducted a survey of Motorway Service Areas by AA Inspectors in order to assess the quality of the facilities they offer for disabled travellers. The tables which follow give updated details of facilities as independently assessed by the Motoring Services Area Management. The information is arranged in numerical order of Motorway, junction by junction.

The aim is to provide sufficient information to enable a disabled motorist to use the motorway network with confidence. Many Motorway Service Areas now use the Service Call System which enables the motorist who needs assistance to alert the staff by means of a call unit which can be purchased in most forecourt shops.

We have made every effort to ensure that the information is up-to-date, but we are dependent on the operators updating any information which may have changed since the inspections took place.

ABBREVIATIONS:

A	=	Fully accessible by wheelchair
NA	=	Not accessible by wheelchair
LIMITED	=	Limited opening times: normally 07.00 - 23.00 or seasonal.
TELEPHONE	=	Height 1.2 metres or less.
UNISEX	=	Own entrance – open 24 hrs unless specified.
WIDE	=	At least 3.6m and suitable for wheelchair.
STANDARD	=	Less than 3.6m and may not be suitable for wheelchair.
DISTANCES	=	Are those from disabled car parking bay to the facility. Distances given – eg 55m – are in metres.

Motorway	Service Area	Parking	Ease of Access	Refreshments	Toilets	Shop	Telephone	Fuel
A1 (M) A195-A69	Washington Northbound Granada (closed Oct-Mar)	2 Spaces wide signed & marked	Fair ramp	10M – A Limited	15M – A Unisex	A Limited space	A internal	Help provided Service call
A1 (M) A195-A69	Washington Southbound Granada	6 Spaces standard signed & marked	Good	10M – A	20M – A Unisex	A	A Disabled internal phone	Help provided Service call
A1 (M)	Gonerby Moor Roundabout Grantham both directions Welcome Break	4 Spaces standard signed & marked	Good	40M – A Restaurant	20M – A Unisex	A	A	Help provided
A1 (M)	Blyth Granada	4 Spaces wide signed & marked	Good	20M – A	20M – A	A	NA	Help provided Service call
M1 Junction 2	Scratchwood Welcome Break	7 Spaces standard signed & marked	Poor steep ramp, heavy doors	55M – A heavy doors	20M – A	A	NA	Help provided
M1 Junction 11-12	Toddington Northbound Granada	4 Spaces wide signed & marked	Fair heavy doors	20-50M – A heavy doors & ramp	20-50M – A Unisex	Poor Steep ramp	NA	Help provided Service call
M1 Junction 12-11	Toddington Southbound Granada	7 Spaces 4 wide 3 standard signed & marked	Good	20-50M – A via lift	20M – A	A	A	Help provided Service call
M1 Junction 14-15	Newport Pagnell Northbound Welcome Break	8 Spaces wide & signed	Poor heavy doors, ramp	40M – A Restaurant heavy doors	A heavy doors	A	NA	Help provided
M1 Junction 15-14	Newport Pagnell Southbound Welcome Break	5 Spaces 3 wide 2 standard signed & marked	Fair steep ramp	20M – A	27M – A	A limited	NA	Help provided
M1 Junction 15-16	Rothersthorpe Northbound Blue Boar	2 Spaces signed & marked	Fair ramp	35M – A Coffee-shop only	35M – A Unisex	A	A	Service call
M1 Junction 16-15	Rothersthorpe Southbound Blue Boar	4 Spaces wide signed & marked	Poor awkward slope	Restaurant upstairs Help provided	40M – A Unisex	A	A	Service call

Motorway	Service Area	Parking	Ease of Access	Refreshments	Toilets	Shop	Telephone	Fuel
A1/A66	**Scotch Corner** Roadside Services Ltd	2 Spaces standard signed & marked	Good	20M Restbite only	25M RADAR key	A	A	Help provided
A1/A46/ A17	**Newark** Roadside Services Ltd	3 Spaces wide marked	Good	30M – A	50M – A	A	A	Help provided
M1 Junction 16-17	**Watford Gap** Northbound Blue Boar	2 Spaces standard signed & marked	Good	40M – A	40M – A Unisex	A	A	Service call
M1 Junction 17-16	**Watford Gap** Southbound Blue Boar	2 Spaces standard signed & marked	Fair ramp	40M – A	40M – A Unisex	A	A	Service call
M1 Junction 21-22	**Leicester Forest East** Northbound Welcome Break	5 Spaces	Good	30M – Fast food	30M – A	A	A	Help provided
M1 Junction 22-21	**Leicester Forest East** Southbound Welcome Break	5 Spaces	Good	30M – Fast food	30M – A	A	A	Help provided
M1 Junction 25-26	**Trowell** Northbound Granada	4 Spaces wide signed & marked	Good	50M – A via lift	25M – A Service call	A	A	Help provided Service call
M1 Junction 26-25	**Trowell** Southbound Granada	3 Spaces wide signed & marked	Good	80M – A	80M – A Service call	A	A	Help provided Service call
M1 Junction 30-31	**Woodall** Northbound Welcome Break	16 Spaces standard signed & marked	Good ramp	41M – A	41M – A Unisex	A	A	Help provided
M1 Junction 31-30	**Woodall** Southbound Welcome Break	11 Spaces standard signed & marked	Good ramp	54M – A	41M – A Unisex	A	A	Help provided
M1 Junction 38-39	**Woolley Edge** Northbound Granada	4 Spaces wide signed & marked	Good	35M – A	35M – A	A restricted	NA	Help provided Service call

Motorway	Service Area	Parking	Ease of Access	Refreshments	Toilets	Shop	Telephone	Fuel
M1 Junction 39-38	**Woolley Edge** Southbound Granada	3 Spaces wide signed & marked	Good	19M – A	25M – A steep ramp	A restricted	NA	Help provided Service call
M2 Junction 4-5	**Farthing Corner** Eastbound Roadside Services Ltd	7 Spaces 3 wide 4 standard signed & marked	Fair ramp	60M – A	110M – A RADAR key	A	A	Help provided
M2 Junction 5-4	**Farthing Corner** Westbound Roadside Services Ltd	8 Spaces 3 wide 5 standard signed & marked	Fair ramp	110M – A	70M – A RADAR key	A	A	Help provided
M3 Junction 5-4	**Fleet** Eastbound Welcome Break	6 Spaces	Fair steep ramps	40M – A	60M – A Unisex	A	A	Help provided
M3 Junction 4-5	**Fleet** Westbound Welcome Break	8 Spaces standard marked	Fair steep ramps	60M – A	73M – A Unisex	NA	A	Help provided Service call
M4 Junction 3-2	**Heston** Eastbound Granada	5 Spaces standard signed & marked	Good	50M – A heavy doors	50M – A Unisex	A	NA	Help provided Service call
M4 Junction 2-3	**Heston** Westbound Granada	6 Spaces standard signed & marked	Good	80M – A heavy doors	80M – A Unisex	A	NA	Help provided Service call
M4 Junction 13	**Chieveley** Granada	5 Spaces – wide poorly signed & marked	Good drop kerbs fitted	50M – A heavy doors	50M – A	A	A	Help provided Service call
M4 Junction 15-14	**Membury** Eastbound Welcome Break	3 Spaces standard signed & marked	Poor heavy doors	80M – A Restaurant via lift Fast food	80M – A	A	A	Help provided
M4 Junction 14-15	**Membury** Westbound Welcome Break	4 Spaces standard signed & marked	Fair heavy doors	100M – A Restaurant via steep access ramp – Fast food	50M – A Unisex	A	A	Help provided
M4 Junction 18-17	**Leigh Delamere** Eastbound Granada	6 Spaces standard signed & marked	Fair heavy doors	50M – A	45M – A Unisex service call	A	NA	Help provided Service call

Motorway	Service Area	Parking	Ease of Access	Refreshments	Toilets	Shop	Telephone	Fuel
M4 Junction 17-18	**Leigh Delamere** Westbound Granada	3 Spaces standard signed & marked	Fair heavy doors	24M – A	46M – A Unisex service call	A	NA	Help provided Service call
M4 Junction 21	**Aust** Roadside Services Ltd	6 Spaces wide signed & marked	Good	40M – A Fast food only Restaurant – lift	45M – A RADAR key	A	A	Help provided
M4 Junction 33	**Cardiff West** Roadside Services Ltd	4 Spaces wide signed & marked	Good	70M – A	45M – A RADAR key	A	A	Help provided
M4 Junction 36	**Sarn Park** Welcome Break	8 Spaces standard marked	Fair spiral ramp	40-47M – A via ramp	37M – A Unisex	A	NA	Help provided 0800-2000
M4 Junction 47	**Swansea** Roadside Services Ltd	4 Spaces wide marked	Good	40M	45M RADAR key	A	A	Help provided
M4 Junction 49	**Pont Abraham** Road Chef	5 Spaces 3 wide 2 standard	Fair heavy doors	31M – A heavy doors	36M – A Unisex	A	A	Help provided 0900-2100
M5 Junction 4-3	**Frankley** Northbound Granada	4 Spaces 2 wide 2 standard marked	Good	20M – A Fast food	20M – A Unisex	A ramp	A	Help provided Service call
M5 Junction 3-4	**Frankley** Southbound Granada	4 Spaces 2 wide 2 standard marked	Poor ramps	40M – A via lift and ramp (through kitchen)	20M – A Unisex	A ramp	A	Help provided Service call
M5 Junction 8-7	**Strensham** Northbound Kenning	16 Spaces wide	Good	30M – A Fast food 60M – A Restaurant	30M – A Unisex	A	A	Help provided
M5 Junction 7-8	**Strensham** Southbound Kenning	3 Spaces standard marked	Poor ramp	50M – A Cafeteria	12M – A Unisex	A	A	Help provided
M5 Junction 14-13	**Michaelwood** Northbound Welcome Break	7 Spaces wide signed & marked	Fair heavy doors	A	75M – A Unisex	A	A	Help provided

Motorway	Service Area	Parking	Ease of Access	Refreshments	Toilets	Shop	Telephone	Fuel
M5 Junction 13-14	**Michaelwood** Southbound Welcome Break	7 Spaces wide signed & marked	Fair heavy doors	A	80M – A Unisex	A	A	Help provided
M5 Junction 19	**Gordano** Welcome Break	7 Spaces wide signed & marked	Fair ramp	25M – A heavy doors	35M – A Unisex difficult	A restricted	A	Help provided
M5 Junction 22-21	**Sedgemoor** Northbound Trust House Forte	4 Spaces standard poorly signed	Good ramp	26M – A	40M – A Unisex limited	A limited	A	Help provided
M5 Junction 21-22	**Sedgemoor** Southbound Road Chef	3 Spaces standard signed & marked	Fair heavy doors	49M – A heavy doors	64M – A Unisex	A	A	Help provided
M5 Junction 26-25	**Taunton Deane** Northbound Road Chef	5/6 Spaces wide signed & marked	Fair heavy doors	75M – A heavy doors limited	75M – A Unisex limited	A limited	A	Help provided 0700-2300
M5 Junction 25-26	**Taunton Deane** Southbound Road Chef	4 Spaces wide signed & marked	Fair heavy doors	61M – A heavy doors	51M – A Unisex	A	A	Help provided
M5 Junction 30	**Exeter** Granada	6 Spaces 1 wide 5 standard signed & marked	Fair heavy doors	88M – A	36M – A Unisex	A	A	Help provided Service call
M6 Junction 3-4	**Corley** Northbound Welcome Break	7 Spaces standard signed & marked	Good	60M – A limited	60M – A Unisex*	A restricted	A	Help provided
M6 Junction 4-3	**Corley** Southbound Welcome Break	6 Spaces standard signed & marked	Good	90M – A	90M – A Unisex*	A restricted	NA	Help provided
M6 Junction 10A-11	**Hilton Park** Northbound Roadside Services Ltd	4 Spaces 2 standard 2 wide signed & marked	Fair ramp	30M – A	60M – A RADAR key	A	A	Help provided
M6 Junction 11-10A	**Hilton Park** Southbound Roadside Services Ltd	8 Spaces 6 standard 2 wide signed & marked	Good	30M – A	50M – A RADAR key	A	A	Help provided

* Key with manager 23.00-06.00

Motorway	Service Area	Parking	Ease of Access	Refreshments	Toilets	Shop	Telephone	Fuel
M6 Junction 15-16	**Keele** Northbound Welcome Break	8 Spaces standard signed & marked	Good automatic doors	30M – A Fast food only	30M – A Unisex*	A	A	Help provided
M6 Junction 15-16	**Keele** Southbound Welcome Break	11 Spaces standard signed & marked	Good	30M – A Fast food only limited	30M – A Unisex*	NA	A	Help provided
M6 Junction 16-17	**Sandbach** Northbound Road Chef	3 Spaces wide signed & marked	Good	45M – A	45M – A Unisex	A	A	Help provided
M6 Junction 17-16	**Sandbach** Southbound Road Chef	3 Spaces wide signed & marked	Good	45M – A	45M – A Unisex	A	A	Help provided
M6 Junction 18-19	**Knutsford** Northbound Roadside Services Ltd	3 Spaces wide signed & marked	Fair ramp	20M – A Fast food only	40M – A RADAR key	A	A	Help provided
M6 Junction 19-18	**Knutsford** Southbound Roadside Services Ltd	4 Spaces wide signed & marked	Fair ramp	20M – A Fast food only	20M – A RADAR key	A	A	Help provided
M6 Junction 27-28	**Charnock Richard** Northbound Welcome Break	10 Spaces wide marked	Good 2 ramps	10M – A Fast food 20M-Restaurant	Adjacent – A Unisex	A	A	Help provided
M6 Junction 28-27	**Charnock Richard** Southbound Welcome Break	10 Spaces wide marked	Good 2 ramps	10M – A Fast food 20M-Restaurant	Adjacent – A Unisex	A	A	Help provided
M6 Junction 32-33	**Forton** Northbound Roadside Services Ltd	4 Spaces wide signed & marked	Good	50M – A Fast food only Restaurant. Lift	50M – A RADAR key	A	A	Help provided
M6 Junction 33-32	**Forton** Southbound Roadside Services Ltd	6 Spaces standard signed & marked	Good ramp	25M – A Fast food only	30M – A RADAR key	A	A	Help provided
M6 Junction 35-36	**Burton** Northbound only Granada	3 Spaces standard signed & marked	Good ramp	20M – A	25M – A 1 Unisex	A Limited space	NA	Help provided Service call

114

Motorway	Service Area	Parking	Ease of Access	Refreshments	Toilets	Shop	Telephone	Fuel
M6 Junction 37-36	**Killington Lake** Southbound only Road Chef	4 Spaces wide signed & marked	Good	20M – A	15M – A 2 (in ladies/gents)	A	A	Help provided 0700-2300
M6 Junction 38-39	**Tebay (West)** Northbound only Westmorland	5 Spaces standard signed & marked	Fair	15M – A	20M – A Unisex	A restricted	A	Help provided
M6 Junction 41-42	**Southwaite** Northbound Granada (7am-11pm)	3 Spaces signed & marked	Good ramp	20M – A	10M – A Unisex	A	A	Service call Help provided
M6 Junction 42-41	**Southwaite** Southbound Granada	4 Spaces signed & marked	Good ramp	50M – A Disabled table	50M – A Unisex	A	A	Service call Help provided
M8 Junction 5-4	**Harthill** Eastbound Road Chef	2 Spaces standard signed & marked	Good ramp	70M – A	84M – A Unisex Key from shop	A	A	Help provided
M8 Junction 4-5	**Harthill** Westbound Road Chef	None	–	Available in forecourt	A Unisex at fuel point	A	Available in forecourt	Help provided
M25 Junction 23	**South Mimms** Welcome Break	8 Spaces wide marked	Fair ramps, heavy doors & raised rail	A 30M – Fast food 85M – Restaurant	55M – A Unisex	A	A	Help scheme Service call
M25 Junction 30-31	**Thurrock** Granada	5 Spaces standard signed & marked	Good	80M – A	80M – A Unisex 2 disabled toilets	A	A	Help provided Service call
M27 Junction 4-3	**Rownhams** Eastbound Road Chef	3 Spaces wide signed & marked	Good heavy doors	50M – A	50M – A Unisex	A	A	Help provided
M27 Junction 3-4	**Rownhams** Westbound Road Chef	1 Space in lorry park wide signed & marked	Good ramp	50M – A	50M – A Unisex	A	A	Help provided
M42 Junction 10	**Tamworth** Granada	5 Spaces standard signed & marked	Good	80M – A	30M – A Unisex disabled toilet	A Ramp	NA	Help provided Service call

Motorway	Service Area	Parking	Ease of Access	Refreshments	Toilets	Shop	Telephone	Fuel
M61 Junction 6-8	**Anderton** Northbound Roadside Services Ltd	3 Spaces wide marked	Fair ramp	50M – A	80M – A RADAR key	A	A	Help provided
M61 Junction 8-6	**Anderton** Southbound Roadside Services Ltd	2 Spaces standard marked	Good ramp	50M – A	50M – A RADAR key	A	A	Help provided
M62 Junction 7-9	**Burtonwood** Eastbound Welcome Break	3 Spaces standard signed & marked	Good ramp	50M – A Little Chef	50M – A Unisex and in garage area	A limited	A	Help provided
M62 Junction 9-7	**Burtonwood** Westbound Welcome Break	3 Spaces standard signed & marked	Fair ramp	50M – A heavy doors	50M – A Unisex in garage area	A (access from E/B side) restricted	A	Help provided
M62 Junction 18-19	**Birch** Eastbound Granada	4 Spaces standard signed & marked	Good	35M – A	Unisex	A	A	Help provided Service call
M62 Junction 19-18	**Birch** Westbound Granada	4 Spaces standard signed & marked	Good	25M – A Disabled table Seasonal	35M – A Unisex	A	A	Help provided Service call
M62 Junction 25-26	**Hartshead Moor** Eastbound Welcome Break	3 Spaces standard signed & marked	Poor steep ramp, heavy doors	A (steep ramp) 57M – Restaurant	29M – A Unisex via Ladies room	A	A	Help provided
M62 Junction 26-25	**Hartshead Moor** Westbound Welcome Break	3 Spaces standard signed & marked	Fair steep ramp	A (steep ramp) 57M – Restaurant	29M – A Unisex via Ladies room	A	A	Help provided
M62 Junction 33	**Ferrybridge** Granada	6 Spaces standard	Good	15M – A disabled table	Unisex Service call	A limited space	A disabled internal phone	Help provided Service call
M74 Junction 4-5	**Hamilton** Northbound only Road Chef	4 Spaces standard signed & marked	Good ramp	30M – A	50M – A Unisex	A	A	Help provided
M74 Junction 6-5	**Bothwell** Southbound only Road Chef	3 Spaces wide signed & marked	Fair heavy doors	30M – A	30M – A Unisex	A	A	Help provided

Motorway	Service Area	Parking	Ease of Access	Refreshments	Toilets	Shop	Telephone	Fuel
M80 Junction 9	**Stirling** All directions Granada	4 Spaces 3 wide 1 standard signed and marked	Good	40M – A	Unisex	A limited space	A disabled external phone	Help provided Service call
M90 Junction 6	**Kinross** Both directions Granada	3 Spaces standard signed & marked	Good ramps	15M – A	Unisex	A not restricted	A	Help provided Service call

THE ORANGE BADGE SCHEME OF PARKING CONCESSIONS FOR DISABLED AND BLIND PEOPLE

The Orange Badge Scheme provides a national system of parking concessions for people with severe disabilities who travel either as drivers or passengers, and for registered blind people. It allows Badge holders to park closer to their destination. In England and Wales you can get an application form and explanatory leaflet about the Scheme from the Social Services Department of your local County, Metropolitan District or London Borough Council. In Scotland you should apply to the Chief Executive of your local Regional or Island Council.

You will qualify for an Orange Badge if you:

(i) receive the higher rate of the mobility component of the Disability Living Allowance
(ii) are registered blind
(iii) use a vehicle supplied by a Government Department *or* get a grant towards your own vehicle
(iv) receive a War Pensioners' Mobility Supplement
(v) have a permanent and substantial disability which causes you very considerable difficulty in walking. In this case your doctor may be asked to provide confirmation of your disability. People with a mental disorder will not normally qualify unless their handicap causes very considerable difficulty in walking
(vi) have a severe disability in both upper limbs, regularly drive a motor vehicle but cannot turn the steering wheel of a motor vehicle by hand even if that wheel is fitted with a turning knob.

The Scheme does not apply in the City of London, the City of Westminster, the Royal Borough of Kensington and Chelsea and part of the London Borough of Camden where there are acute parking problems. These authorities run their own schemes for people living and working in their area. In addition, the Scheme does not apply at some airports (eg Heathrow), and access to certain town centres may be prohibited or limited to vehicles with special permits. With these exceptions, the Orange Badge Scheme applies throughout England, Scotland and Wales.

Badge holders may park free of charge and without time limit at on-street parking meters, "pay and display" on-street parking and in time-limited waiting areas. Badge holders may also park on single or double yellow lines for up to three hours in England and Wales and without time limit in Scotland, except where there is a ban on loading and unloading.

In England and Wales you will also need a special parking disc, in addition to the Orange Badge, when you park on yellow lines. People with disabilities living in Scotland who wish to visit England and Wales should be able to get this disc from their local Regional or Island Council.

The Orange Badge is not a licence to park anywhere, and Badge holders have the same obligations as other road users to ensure that they park safely and do not cause an obstruction. Vehicles which are parked dangerously or obstructively can be removed by the police.

Misuse of a Badge may lead to it being withdrawn. It is also illegal for able-bodied people to use a Badge. If they do so they are liable to a fine of up to £1,000.

Some other European countries allow disabled visitors to take advantage of the parking concessions provided for their own citizens by displaying the Orange Badge (see page 140). Further details of these benefits may be obtained by writing to the Department of Transport, Room C10/02, 2 Marsham Street, London SW1P 3EB.

NORTHERN IRELAND

The Department of the Environment for Northern Ireland operates an Orange Badge Scheme similar to that in England and Wales under the Chronically Sick and Disabled Persons (Northern Ireland) Act 1978.

Applications should be made to the appropriate Roads Service Division of the Department of the Environment. Security restrictions on parking in urban areas will inevitably limit the scope of the concessions.

JERSEY

The States of Jersey also have an Orange Badge Scheme, issued on grounds very similar to those in the United Kingdom and for that reason United Kingdom issued Badges are accepted. However, the regulations are different and details must be obtained from the Town Hall, St Helier, Jersey, Channel Islands.

EXEMPTION FROM PAYMENT OF VEHICLE EXCISE DUTY FOR DISABLED PEOPLE

Disabled people who are in receipt of the higher rate of the mobility component of Disability Living Allowance or War Pensioners' Mobility Supplement are eligible to apply for a Vehicle Excise Duty Exemption Certificate.

Invalid carriages are exempt from vehicle excise duty; the vehicle must be registered in the name of the disabled person and used solely by or for the purposes of the disabled person. For advice contact: Department of Transport, Vehicle Standards and Engineering, 2 Marsham Street, London SW1P 3EB.

Disabled people who are in receipt of Attendance Allowance or a care component of Disability Living Allowance may be entitled to exemption from Vehicle Excise Duty. To qualify for the exemption he/she must be cared for and driven by a full-time constant attendant and satisfy certain mobility requirements. The vehicle must be registered in the name of the disabled person (special arrangements about registration apply for a child).

Application for exemption should be made to:

1 **Disability Living Allowance with the higher rate of the mobility component**
Disability Living Allowance Unit, Warbreck House, Warbreck Hill, Blackpool FY2 0TE *tel* (0345) 123456.

2 **War Pensioners Mobility Supplement**
WPMS Section, Norcross, Blackpool FY5 3TA *tel* (0253) 856123.

3 **Attendance Allowance or Disability Living Allowance: the care component**
DLA Unit (IVS Section), Warbreck House, Warbreck Hill, Blackpool FY2 0TE *tel* (0345) 123456.

A leaflet V188 Exemption from Vehicle Excise Duty for Disabled People is available from the DVLC Swansea.

DISABILITY LIVING ALLOWANCE

Disability Living Allowance is a benefit for people who need help with getting around, help with personal care or help with both of these. There are fixed amounts of money for help with getting around and for help with personal care; if you need help with both you can normally get both amounts of money.

The allowance may be claimed by disabled people aged between 5 and under 66 years (if you are already 65, you will have to show that you could have qualified for the allowance immediately before you were 65).

Further information and a claim pack can be obtained from all Department of Social Security Offices and there is a free Benefit Enquiry Line *tel* 0800-882 200.

MOTABILITY

Motability is incorporated by Royal Charter and a registered charity which was set up with the support of the Government. Its aim is to help people with a mobility allowance and War Pensioners' Mobility Supplement to use their allowance/Supplement to obtain a car or powered wheelchair. Over 200,000 vehicles have already been provided through the scheme.

New cars can be obtained either on hire for 3 years or by hire purchase. Under the hire scheme there are a variety of models available, including the Rover Group, Citroen, Fiat, Ford, Nissan, Peugeot, Proton, Renault, Toyota, Vauxhall, Volkswagen and Volvo; servicing and maintenance, AA membership and loss-of-use insurance cover are included. For the hire purchase scheme, special discounts have been negotiated with the mentioned manufacturers but virtually any make can be purchased over 5 years. Additionally there are hire purchase schemes for used cars and powered wheelchairs.

For all schemes, disabled people agree to the Department of Social Security paying this allowance or Supplement to Motability Finance Ltd (MFL) for the period of their agreement. MFL was set up by the Clearing Banks to serve only Motability customers, and finance is made available at preferential interest rates.

Motability's charitable funds are used to help

customers who need financial assistance to meet the cost of initial deposits and any special adaptions. Further information is available from Motability, Gate House, West Gate, Harlow, Essex, CM20 1HR *tel* Harlow (0279) 635666 (Helpline).

SEAT BELT REGULATIONS – MEDICAL EXEMPTIONS

Regulations concerning the compulsory wearing of seat belts when travelling in the front seat of cars and light vans came into force on 31 January 1983. Further regulations were introduced concerning children in rear seats on 1st July 1989, and adults in rear seats on 1st July 1991. Medical exemptions can apply to all seats.

In its leaflet 'Seat Belts, the Law and You' the Department of Transport gives hints and guidance on all aspects of the seat belt law. This includes an explanation of the requirements and procedures to apply for a medical exemption certificate and incorporates a form which has to be completed if you are to obtain a free medical examination. The leaflet can be obtained from the Department of Transport, Room C18/12 Marsham Street, London SW1P 3EB *tel* 071-276 0800.

PRINCIPAL TOLL BRIDGES AND TUNNELS

Disabled drivers using the toll bridges and tunnels listed on the next page may be entitled to concessions provided they meet certain requirements. In most cases to qualify for a concession an application has to be made in advance to the relevant bridge/tunnel or local authority. This may well preclude the casual visitor from qualifying for a concession so please check the situation first.

MOTORWAY REGULATIONS AND THE DISABLED DRIVER

Drivers of invalid carriages and tricycles are sometimes in doubt as to whether or not such vehicles are allowed on motorways.

The 1988 Road Traffic Act section 185 clearly defines an invalid carriage as a mechanically propelled vehicle that is specially designed and constructed, and not merely adapted, for the disabled, and which does not exceed 254 kgs (5 cwt) unladen. Such a vehicle is not allowed on motorways.

Ordinary motor cars that have been adapted for a disabled person are permitted on motorways.

Invalid tricycles and vehicles specially designed and constructed for disabled people are permitted on motorways provided that they weigh more than 254 kgs (5 cwt). Invalid tricycles are no longer being issued to disabled persons by the DHSS.

USE OF INVALID CARRIAGES ON PAVEMENTS

Regulations permit the use of small powered invalid pavement carriages (unladen weight 250 lb or less), which are incapable of exceeding four miles per hour, on public pavements. Carriages so used must have an efficient braking system.

BREAKDOWN ASSISTANCE

24-hour AA Breakdown Service for the disabled The full range of benefits of AA Membership is open to drivers of single-seater, motor-propelled, three-wheeled invalid carriages through a special membership at the annual subscription of £10 which includes Relay, Relay Plus and Home Start Services (the £10 joining fee is not charged).

Converted four-wheelers can only be accepted under the normal conditions of Personal Membership, regardless of how they are classified by the authorities. However, if the car has been obtained through the Motability scheme (*see page 119*) then the £10 joining fee only, will not be charged.

Benefits of Personal Membership include 24-hour Roadside Service by AA Patrols or AA-appointed garages (for full details see the *AA Members' Handbook*) with the option to take out Relay, Relay Plus and Homestart.

If a prompt repair cannot be arranged locally, following a roadside breakdown, accident, or act of vandalism, Relay provides for recovery of the vehicle and transportation of it, together with the driver (and up to four passengers in the case of a converted four-wheeler) to any single destination in the British Isles. (Relay does not operate in the Republic of Ireland.)

Continued on page 122

BRIDGES

Clifton Bridge	(B3124 W of Bristol)	Exemption for recipients of mobility allowance on prior application for annual season tickets (50p) subject to satisfactory documentary proof from: Coopers & Lybrand, 66 Queen Square, Bristol BS1 4JP.
Dartford Bridge	(River Thames)	Exemption from payment of Vehicle Excise Duty qualifies.
Dunham Bridge	(A57 Lincoln – Worksop)	Ministry supplied, hand-controlled vehicles only.
Erskine Bridge	(nr Glasgow)	Exempt.
Forth Bridge	(nr Edinburgh)	Exemption for holders of an Orange Badge (Disabled person must be travelling in vehicle).
Humber Bridge	(nr Hull)	Exemption on prior application for tickets to holders of tax exemption certificates MY 182, MHS 330, MPB 1266 and also drivers of Invehcars. Address: Humber Bridge Board, Administration Building, Ferriby Road, Hessle, North Humberside HU13 0JG.
Itchen Bridge	(A3025 Woolston – Southampton)	Motor cycle, invalid carriage or disabled persons vehicle – reduced toll charge of 10p.
Porthmadog	(A487, E of town)	Exempt.
Severn Bridge	(M4 Aust, nr Bristol/Chepstow)	Exemption for holders of an Orange Badge. Allowed free passage.
Tamar Bridge	(A38 Plymouth – Liskeard)	Exemption for registered blind persons and recipients of disability living allowance with mobility component at the higher level. Send stamped addressed envelope for voucher application form to The Manager, Tamar Bridge & Torpoint Ferry, 2 Ferry Street, Torpoint, Cornwall PL11 2AX.
Tay Bridge	(Newport – Dundee)	Exempt.
Whitchurch Bridge	(B471 Pangbourne – Whitchurch)	Exempt. (Disabled person must be travelling in vehicle.

TUNNELS

Dartford Tunnel	(River Thames)	Exemption from payment of Vehicle Excise Duty qualifies.
Mersey Tunnel	(Liverpool – Birkenhead – Wallasey)	Details on application to: The General Manager, Mersey Tunnels, Georges Dock Building, Georges Dock Way, Pier Head, Liverpool L3 1DD.
Tyne Tunnel	(nr Newcastle)	Exemption from payment of Vehicle Excise Duty qualifies.

Relay Plus is an optional extension of Relay, and enables the member to have 48 hours use of a hire car, or overnight accommodation (up to five persons), or re-imbursement of public transport costs.

Home Start extends the 24-hour Roadside Service to the Member's home. If the car cannot be repaired promptly, the AA will arrange for it to be towed to the nearest AA-appointed garage, or other local destination.

All Orange Badge holders and profoundly deaf motorists are entitled to a special discount on 'Comprehensive Membership' – Personal, Relay and Home Start taken together. This offer is open to both new and existing members. For further details please contact Bristol (0272) 251519.

AA Disabled Helpline

A new service for the Disabled Motorist. Call free on 0800 262 050 for free information and advice, to join the AA or to renew Membership, or when you need breakdown assistance if you are already an AA Member.

Callsafe

The AA's innovative Callsafe emergency phone system allows motorists to call for breakdown assistance or the emergency services, including the police, without leaving the car. The system is powered either from the cigarette lighter socket of a battery power pack.

AA Callsafe costs £199 for the equipment, with a one-off £35.25 network joining fee. Thereafter, users pay only the quarterly subscriptions of £29.99 for access to the cellular phone system.

'Keep Mobile' Alternative Transport Costs for Disabled Motorists

AA Insurance Services have developed an insurance policy tailor-made to suit the individual needs of the physically disabled motorist to keep them on the move when their cars are off the road for repair as a result of an accident. Whether it be a specially adapted vehicle or a vehicle registered and insured in your name but driven for you by a nominated driver, the Disabled Motorists' Loss of Use Policy could take away a lot of the worry by providing cover for those extra expenses.

Under the scheme you could cover the daily cost of train, bus or taxi fares, or if you prefer, you can hire a vehicle. AA Insurance has made arrangements with Hertz Rent-A-Car to provide for hire of a vehicle, adapted to hand controls, to accommodate drivers with lower limb disabilities, which can normally be made available with 24 hours notice. Or, if you are not a driver yourself but have someone to drive on your behalf due to your disability, then you too will qualify to hire a car from Hertz.

To qualify for the scheme it is necessary for you to have arranged comprehensive cover through AA Insurance and to have notified the DVLC of your disability. Quotations can be obtained at any of the 250 AA shops, or by dialling 100 and asking for Freefone AA Autoquote.

Hearing-impaired motorists who break down at the roadside can now contact the AA directly using the Association's nationwide service for Minicom users. By dialling the AA's free national breakdown number 0800 887766, deaf callers with a Minicom visual display telephone can type and transmit their details to the nearest AA Operations Centre. Trained Minicom operators are able to type back an answer and quickly arrange for assistance. The Minicom telephone can be purchased from Teletec International, Sunningdale House, 49 Caldecotte Business Park, Milton Keynes MK7 8LF *tel* (0908) 270003 *Minicom* (0908) 270005

AA/RAC assistance cards

These are issued by the branch of the Ministry of Social Security responsible for providing vehicles and allowances to disabled war veterans. They are available only to war veterans, provided that the vehicle used has been issued by the Ministry under the special arrangements.

These cards are free and persons holding them are entitled to AA and RAC patrol assistance in an emergency. The ownership of a card does not, however, entitle the holder to any other benefits; if these are required, Membership should be taken out in the appropriate class. (See page 120.)

For further information contact: Department of Social Security, North Fylde Central Office, Norcross, Blackpool FY5 3TA *tel* (0253) 856123 ext 63222 (War Pensions), ext 67277 (Invalid Vehicle Scheme).

REPAIR OF INVALID CHAIRS AND THREE-WHEELERS

Owners of three-wheelers and Government issue four-wheeled cars in need of repair should contact their local repairer or DLA (I.V.S) Room C309, Fylde Benefits and War Pensions Directorate, Warbreck House, Warbreck Hill Road, Blackpool FY5 3TA *tel* (0253) 754137/8. For other invalid chairs and wheelchairs contact your local hospital.

SELF-DRIVE HIRE

Wheelchair Travel Ltd is a new self-drive rental company which offers the hire of wheelchair adapted minibuses for any period for UK or continental travel. All their vehicles are equipped with tail-lifts, floor clamps, and full inertia reel harness. Rear seat belts, PA, stereo radio/cassette and vehicle security alarm. Each vehicle will carry up to two wheelchairs, and 6 to 8 able-bodied. Rates include comprehensive insurance cover for UK, as well as non-UK, licence holders. For information and bookings contact: Wheelchair Travel, 1 Johnston Green, Guildford, Surrey GU2 6XS *tel* (0483) 233640.

'HELP' PENNANT

A very effective 'help' pennant which a stranded disabled motorist can attach to his/her car window to attract attention has been developed by the Department of Transport. This can be useful not just if your car breaks down, but, for example, at petrol stations as well.

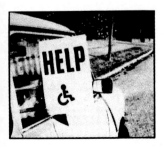

They cost £5 including postage and packing. Available from G.P. Special Products Ltd, 69 West Hill, Portishead, Bristol BS20 9LG *tel* (0275) 842322.

TRAVELLING ON BRITISH RAIL

British Rail are able to offer a number of services, all of which are completely free to disabled travellers and are to be found in the leaflet 'British Rail and Disabled Travellers'. If notified in advance (a couple of days notice should suffice) arrangements can be made to ensure your trip is as comfortable as possible. Special arrangements can be made at departure and destination points, and at any intermediate stations where travellers need to change trains, to safely escort the disabled traveller. The local Area Manager at the departure station should be notified in this instance.

DISABLED PERSONS RAILCARD

In addition, if you are disabled (in accordance with the provisions shown by British Rail in their leaflet) you may purchase the 'Disabled Persons Railcard'. This allows you, and if you wish, an accompanying adult, both to travel by train with a $33^{1}/_{3}$% discount on Cheap and Standard Day Returns, Standard Single, Return and Saver Fares. Full details of the scheme are outlined in a special leaflet. A Disabled Persons Railcard is valid for 12 months from date of issue. Leaflets and full details of services for the disabled are available from your local BR Station or by contacting British Rail, PO Box 28, York YO1 1FB.

COACH AND BUS TRAVEL

It is now the policy to design new coach stations with wheelchair users in mind and some of the newer stations do have facilities such as accessible toilets and refreshment areas. However, many of the older ones have no wheelchair access. Contact coach stations you may wish to use to find out what facilities are available. Similarly some individual coach companies can accommodate wheelchair users if contacted beforehand. Victoria Coach Station is undergoing refurbishment at the time of going to press and will have improved facilities for disabled people by early 1993. Some help is available but always check in advance of your travel date so that arrangements can be made *tel* 071-730 3466.

London Transport run a Unit for Disabled Passengers which operates special services and provides advice and information regarding routes, Underground stations, trains and concessionary fares. Carelink buses run hourly every day of the year (except 25-26 December). They connect all the London terminus rail stations and link up with Airbus, the wheelchair accessible bus service to Heathrow Airport. For a free information pack *tel* 071-918 3312 (voice and Minicom), or write to: The Unit for Disabled Passengers, London Transport, 55 Broadway, London SW1H 0BD.

COACH TOURS

The following company has available for hire coaches with chairlift. Further information and bookings from: Andrew Miller, 13 Willow Way, Hauxton, Cambridgeshire CB2 5JB *tel* Cambridge (0223) 837030.

HOLIDAYS AT SEA

The 'Jubilee Sailing Trust' is a charity that offers physically disabled adults (aged 16-70) the opportunity to sail as active crew members on a 180′ tall ship. The *Lord Nelson*, their square rigged sailing ship was designed to enable disabled crew members to participate on equal terms with those who are able bodied. She is sailed by forty voyage crew (of whom half are disabled) on voyages lasting from a weekend to ten days.

She sails around the United Kingdom, Channel Islands and Europe from March to November and in the Canary Islands during the winter season.

For further details of how to become a *Lord Nelson* crew member contact: Jubilee Sailing Trust, Test Road, Eastern Docks, Southampton SO1 1GG *tel* (0703) 631395.

HOLIDAY CARE SERVICE

This registered charity is a free information service on holidays for disabled people. The Service holds extensive details of accommodation, transport, guidebooks, inclusive holidays in the United Kingdom and abroad, and possible sources of financial help. They do not make reservations or bookings, but provide as much information as possible from which the enquirer can make a choice. Individuals, their families, friends or those who care for them, can telephone or write, explaining their problem and what kind of holiday they want, where they would like to go, and what sort of budget they have. They provide competitive insurance particularly for elderly and disabled people, their friends and families. For further information contact: Holiday Care Service, 2 Old Bank Chambers, Station Road, Horley, Surrey RH6 9HW *tel* Horley (0293) 774535.

TOILET FACILITIES

Some local authorities are finding it necessary to restrict access to their public conveniences as a means of preventing vandalism and reducing running costs. These authorities have been asked to join the National Key Scheme, whereby a standard lock is fitted and keys are made available to disabled people, either through the local authority or from RADAR.

The scheme is not in use everywhere – unfortunately, a number of local authorities do not have suitable toilets and, more happily, others do not have vandalism problems. This has led to problems with the compiling of comprehensive information, however, should you require further details a book has been compiled by RADAR which gives details of over 3,500 toilets available through the scheme.

For those who are unable to obtain a key in their own locality, RADAR supplies keys at a charge of £2.50 inclusive of postage and packing. A full list of the locations of the toilets is also available for £3.00 inclusive of postage and packaging.

SHOPMOBILITY

Shopmobility is the name being used throughout the UK to describe schemes for people who through disability, illness, accident or advancing age need a manual wheelchair, a power chair or a scooter, to go shopping. The service is generally provided free, though some schemes require a deposit.

Aberdeen Shopmobility
The scheme is open Tuesday-Thursday 10am-4pm, Friday 8.30am-4pm and Saturday 8.30am-1pm. Manual chairs, powered scooters and powered chairs are available.

For further information contact: Shopmobility,

Flowermill Lane, Aberdeen *tel* (0224) 630009.

Basildon Shopmobility
Open Monday-Friday 9am-4pm, manual chairs, powered scooter and powered chairs are available.

For further information contact: 103A Lower Galleries, Eastgate Centre, Basildon, Essex SS41 1AG *tel* (0268) 533644.

Bexleyheath, Broadway Shopping Centre
Bexleyheath Shopmobility can provide assistance to the disabled shopper in the form of wheelchair loan, with electric scooters and electrically powered and hand-propelled chairs, together with the provision of volunteers to push the chair and generally aid the shopper.

The service operates 10am-3pm, Tuesday and Friday. Chairs and volunteers can be booked in advance, in which case the shopper can be met in the car park or Centre entrance. An intercom to the Shopmobility office is situated near the disabled parking places in the car park.

For chair and/or volunteer reservations *tel* 081-301 5237 between 10am-3pm, Tuesday and Friday.

Bradford Shopmobility
The Bradford scheme is open Monday, Tuesday, Thursday and Friday, 9am-5pm, Wednesday and Saturday 9am-1pm. For further details: Shopmobility, John Street Market, Rawson Road, Bradford, West Yorkshire *tel* (0274) 754076.

Braintree Shopmobility
Powered scooters are available Monday-Saturday 9am-4.30pm.

For further details contact: First Shop Centre, Town Hall Annexe, Fairfield Road, Braintree *tel* (0376) 46535.

Brierley Hill, Merryhill Shopping Centre
For information on Brierley Hill Shopmobility: Merryhill Shopping Centre, Brierley Hill, West Midlands DY5 1SY *tel* (0384) 481141. Adjacent to the shopping centre is a superstore selling aids etc. for disabled people. For further information *tel* (0384) 484544.

Cambridge Shopmobility
Open Wednesday, Thursday and Saturday, 10am-4pm. Manual chairs, powered scooters and powered chairs are available at Level 9. Lion Yard Car Park, Cambridge *tel* (0223) 463370. Correspondence to Engineers Dept., Cambridge City Council, The Guildhall, Cambridge.

Cardiff City Centre
Cardiff Shopmobility is a scheme to provide wheelchairs on loan, both power and manual chairs and scooters, extended leg rests and an amputee chair, to disabled persons to allow them to shop and use other facilities in the city centre.

Free reserved parking is available for users of the scheme on the ground floor of the Oxford Arcade Multi-Storey Car Park with a separate access from Bridge Street. After transferring to a wheelchair, disabled shoppers will be able to visit the St Davids Shopping Centre and shops in adjoining Queen Street. The Hayes and St Davids Hall and the covered market. Manual chairs are also available for the longer-stay visitor at a modest charge.

For further information contact The Manager, Shopmobility, Bridge Street, Cardiff CF2 2EB *tel* Cardiff (0222) 399355.

Central Milton Keynes Shopping Centre
By contacting the Centre's Shopmobility service in advance, it is possible to reserve a motorised, or hand-propelled wheelchair which is collected on arrival, on production of proof of identity. After a 'driving lesson' the centre is the handicapped visitor's oyster. Travelling is made easy by the absence of steps and kerbs.

For further information write to CMK Shopping Management Co Ltd, 96 Midsummer Arcade, Secklow Gate West, Central Milton Keynes MK9 3ES.

For wheelchair reservations please telephone: Shopmobility, Shopping Information Unit on Milton Keynes (0908) 670231.

Chesterfield Shopmobility
Open Monday-Saturday, 10am-4pm. Manual chairs, powered scooters and powered chairs are available.

For further information contact: Chesterfield Shopmobility, Ground Floor, Multi-Storey Car Park, New Beetwell Street, Chesterfield, Derbyshire S40 1QR *tel* (0246) 209668.

Chiltern Shopmobility
Open Monday-Friday, 9am-1pm. Powered scooters are available.
For further information contact: The Malthouse, Elgiva Lane, Chesham, Buckinghamshire *tel* (0494) 778400.

Colchester Shopmobility
Open Tuesday-Thursday, 10am-4pm. Manual chairs, powered scooters and powered chairs are available.
For further information contact; 15 Queen Street, Colchester, Essex CO1 2PH *tel* (0206) 369099.

Cwmbran Shopmobility
Open Monday-Friday, 9am-5pm. Manual chairs, powered scooters and powered chairs are available.
For further information contact: 17 Caradoc Road Town Centre, Cwmbran, Gwent *tel* (06333) 62951.

Dartford Shopmobility
Open Monday, Tuesday and Saturday 8am-6pm, Wednesday, Thursday and Friday 8am-8pm.
For further information contact: Priory Shopping Centre, Dartford, Kent DA1 2HS *tel* (0322) 220915.

Derby Shopmobility
Derby Shopmobility is open Monday-Friday, 9.30am-5pm. Free loan of manual wheelchairs and battery powered scooters; instruction will be given on the scooter. Escort assistance also available if required. Free disabled parking in Shopmobility spaces which can be reserved; booking in advance is recommended.
For further information: Derby Shopmobility, The Portacabin, Bold Lane Car Park, Derby DE1 3NT *tel* (0332) 200320.

Dewsbury Shopmobility
Open Monday-Friday, 9am-4pm. Manual chair, powered scooter and powered chair available.
For further details contact: Shopmobility, Town Hall Way, Dewsbury WF12 8EQ *tel* (0924) 455149.

Edinburgh and Lothian
Open Tuesday-Saturday, 10am-4pm. Located at The Mound Centre, Edinburgh 2 *tel* 031-225 9559.

Manual chairs, powered scooters and powered chairs are available.
Correspondence to: LRC King Stables' Yard, King Stables' Road, Edinburgh EH2 2YJ.

Falkirk Shopmobility
Open Monday-Friday, 10.30am-4pm, manual and powered chairs available. On Saturday manual chairs only by arrangement with security guards.
For further details contact: Shopmobility, Howgate Shopping Centre, High Street, Falkirk FK1 1DN *tel*

Gateshead, Metro Centre
Gateshead Shopmobility is open Monday to Wednesday and Friday, 10am-8pm, Thursday 10am-9pm, Saturday 9am-6pm. For further details: Shopmobility, Metro Centre, Gateshead, Tyne & Wear NE11 9YG *tel* 091-460 5299.

Glasgow Shopmobility
Open Monday-Saturday, 10am-4pm. Manual chairs, powered scooters and powered chairs.
For further details contact: Shopmobility, 6th Floor, Sauchiehall Centre, 179 Sauchiehall Street, Glasgow G2 3ER *tel* 041-353 2594.

Gloucester Shopmobility
Open Tuesday-Friday, 9.30am-5pm. Manual chair, powered scooters and powered chairs. Located at Hampden Way, Gloucester.
For further information *tel* (0452) 396898 or write to: The Herbert Warehouse, The Docks, Gloucester GL1 2EQ.

Harlow Shopmobility
The Harlow Shopmobility scheme is open Monday to Saturday. Apr-Sep 9.30am-4pm; Oct-Mar 9.30am-4pm. For further details: Post Office Car Park, Harlow CM20 1AA *tel* (0279) 446188.

Hatfield Shopmobility
Hatfield Shopmobility is open Tuesday to Saturday, 9am-5pm. For further information: Shopmobility, 98 Town Centre, The Commons, Hatfield, Herts AL10 0NG *tel* (0707) 262731.

Hemel Hempstead
Open Tuesday-Saturday, 9.30am-5pm. Manual chairs, powered scooters and powered chairs.

For further details contact: Level A Car Park, Marlowes Shopping Centre, Marlowes, Hemel Hempstead, Herts HP1 1DX *tel* (0442) 259259.

Hereford Shopmobility

The Hereford Shopmobility Centre is situated in the underground car park at the Maylord Orchards shopping complex. Manual wheelchairs, powered wheelchairs and scooters are available for hire at no charge. A map of the central area of Hereford is supplied, with the areas suited to wheelchairs and scooters marked in orange. It is advisable to book in advance and to state your needs.

The service operates Monday to Saturday (ex Bank Hols), 9am-5pm. For further information: Hereford Shopmobility, Maylord Orchards Car Park, Blueschool Street, Hereford *tel* (0432) 342166.

Huddersfield Shopmobility

Open Monday-Friday, 9am-4pm. Manual chairs, powered scooters and powered chairs available.

For further details contact: Disability Services, The Day Centre, Zetland Street, Huddersfield HD1 2RA *tel* (0484) 453000.

Ipswich Shopmobility Centre

The Ipswich scheme is open daily Monday to Saturday, 10.30am-5.30pm. For further details: Upper Barclay Street, Ipswich, Suffolk IP4 1HU *tel* (0473) 222225.

Keighley Shopmobility

The scheme is open Monday, Wednesday, Thursday and Friday, 9am-5pm, Tuesday and Saturday, 9am-1pm. For further details: Shopmobility, Cooke Street, Keighley, West Yorkshire *tel* (0274) 758225.

Kingston-Upon-Thames Shopmobility

The service is open Monday to Saturday, 9am-5pm. Further information: Shopmobility, Eden Walk Car Park, Union Street, Kingston-Upon-Thames KT1 1BL *tel* 081-547 1255.

Kirkcaldy Shopmobility

Open Tuesday 9am-4.15pm, Wednesday and Thursday 1pm-4.15pm, Friday 9.15am-4.15pm. Manual chairs, powered scooters and powered chairs available.

For further details contact: Shopmobility, Mercat Centre Car Park, Tolbooth Street, Kirkcaldy *tel* (0592) 640940.

Leicester Shopmobility

Leicester Shopmobility is open Monday to Friday, 10am-5pm and Saturday, 10am-1pm. For further details: Ground Floor, Newarke Street Car Park, Near The Phoenix, Leicester LE1 6ZG *tel* (0533) 526694.

Lincoln Shopmobility

Open Monday-Saturday, 9am-4pm. Manual chairs available. For further details contact: Shopmobility, Tentercroft Street Car Park, Lincoln *tel* (0522) 544983.

Luton Shopmobility

Open Monday-Saturday, 9.30am-4.30pm. Manual chairs, powered scooters and powered chairs available. Located at Level 3 Market Car Park, Melson Street, Luton.

For further details contact: Arndale Management Office, Unit 37 Arndale Centre, Luton *tel* (0582) 38936.

Newport Shopping Centre

Newport Shopmobility is open Monday to Saturday, 9am-5pm. For further details: Newport Shopmobility, 193 Upper Dock Street, Newport, Gwent NP9 1DA *tel* (0633) 223845.

A shopmobility Newport service also operates from the Kingsway Shopping Centre, Kingsway, Newport, Monday to Saturday, 9am-5pm *tel* (0633) 243688.

Northampton Shopmobility

The service is open Tuesday to Friday, 10am-4pm. Further details: Northampton Shopmobility, 13 Hazlewood Road, Northampton NN1 1LG *tel* (0604) 233714.

Nottingham Shopmobility

The Nottingham scheme is open Monday to Saturday, 9am-5pm. For further information: St Nicholas Centre, Stanford Street, Nottingham NG1 6AE *tel* (0602) 584486.

Peterborough, Queensgate Regional Covered Shopping Centre

Peterborough Shopmobility is a scheme to•

provide electrically powered or hand-propelled wheelchairs or three-wheeled scooters to help people who have limited mobility to shop and use other facilities in the city centre.

The service operates 10am-5pm, Monday to Friday, extended to 7.30pm for late shopping on Thursday and 9am-5pm Saturday.

The scheme is based on the car park connected to Queensgate – the covered shopping centre – which is linked to the city centre's other streets. For further information and to ensure that a chair is available, tel Peterborough (0733) 313133, or write to Peterborough Shopmobility, Queensgate, Peterborough PE1 1NT. If you need any special features or fittings on a chair – ask, they may be available.

Plymouth Shopping Centre
Plymouth Shopmobility offers on FREE loan, within the city centre, electric scooters and electric and manual wheelchairs. Open Monday to Saturday, 9am-5pm. For information on Plymouth Shopmobility: Charles Cross Car Park, Eastlake Street, Plymouth, Devon tel (0752) 600633.

Preston Shopmobility
Open Monday-Friday, 9am-5pm. Manual chairs, powered scooters and powered chairs available.

For further details contact: Shopmobility, 28 Friargate, Preston tel (0772) 204667.

Redbridge Shopmobility
Open Wednesday and Friday, 10am-4pm. Manual chairs, powered scooters and powered chairs. Located at ground level, the Exchange Car Park.

Further details from: The Management Suite, The Exchange Car Park, High Road, Ilford, Essex tel 081-478 6864.

Redditch Shopmobility
Redditch Shopmobility is open Monday to Wednesday and Friday, 9am-6pm, Thursday, 9am-7.30pm and Saturday, 9am-5.30pm. For further details: Kingfisher Centre, Car Park 3, Redditch, Worcs B97 4HL tel (0527) 69922.

Sandwell Shopping Centre
Sandwell Shopmobility is open Monday to Wednesday 9am-5pm, Thursday and Friday

9am-5.30pm, Saturday, 8.30am-4.30pm. For further information: Level One, Multi Storey Car Park, Queens Square, Sandwell Centre, West Bromwich tel 021-553 1943.

Southend on Sea Shopmobility
Open Tuesday and Thursday-Saturday, 10am-4pm. Manual and powered chairs. Located at Farringdon Car Park, off Elmer Approach, Southend on Sea, Essex.

For further details write to: 74 Hampton Gardens, Southend on Sea tel (0702) 339682.

Sutton Shopmobility
Open Tuesday-Saturday, 10am-4pm. Manual chairs, powered scooters and powered chairs available.

For further details contact: Gibson Road Car Park, Sutton, Surrey tel 081-770 0691.

Sutton Coldfield Shopmobility
The scheme is open Monday to Saturday, 9am-5pm. For further information: Gracechurch Shopping Centre, Sutton Coldfield B72 1PH tel 021-355 1112.

Telford Shopping Centre
Telford Shopmobility is open Monday to Thursday 9am-5pm, Friday, 9am-8pm. For further details: Shopmobility, c/o Information Centre, Piccadilly Square, Telford Shopping Centre, Telford tel (0952) 291370.

Wigan Shopmobility
Open Monday-Saturday, 9am-5pm. Manual chairs, powered scooters and powered chairs available.

For further details contact: 1 Wigan Gallery, The Galleries Shopping Centre, Wigan WN1 1AR tel (0942) 825520.

Worcester Shopmobility
The service is open Monay to Saturday, 9am-5pm. Further information: Worcester Shopmobility, 54 Priory Walk, Crowngate Centre, Worcester tel (0905) 610523.

Woking Shopmobility
Open Monday-Friday 9.30am-5pm, also Saturday 9am-5pm. Manual chair, powered scooters and powered chairs available.

For further details contact: The Peacocks, Victoria Way, Woking, Surrey GU21 1CD *tel* (0483) 776612.

Yeovil Shopmobility
Yeovil Shopmobility is open Monday to Friday, 9am-4.30pm. For further details: Petters House, Petters Way, Yeovil, Somerset BA20 1SH *tel* (0935) 75914.

ARTS AND ENTERTAINMENT

Access information for disabled people to art and entertainment venues in the Greater London area is provided by 'Artsline', 5 Crowndale Road, London NW1 1TU. Telephone 071-388 2227 Mon-Fri (9.30am-5.30pm). The Arts and Listings magazine "Disability Arts in London" is available free to disabled people by telephoning or writing to the address above.

USEFUL PUBLICATIONS

Shown below are a selection of the many publications available through RADAR.
For an up-to-date price list write to the Royal Association for Disability and Rehabilitation, 25 Mortimer Street, London W1N 8AB, enclosing a large stamped addressed envelope.

General guides from RADAR
Holidays in the British Isles: a guide for disabled people; Holidays and Travel Abroad: a guide for disabled people; Motoring and Mobility for Disabled People.

Sport and leisure
Guide to sports centres for disabled people; Countryside & Wildlife for disabled people.
Spectators' Access Guide for Disabled People – a regional guide to facilities at sporting venues in England.

Town/City Guides
A guide for London is available and RADAR can give details of over 350 local access guides.

Publications published by the Joint Committee on Mobility for the Disabled and available through RADAR
RADAR Mobility Factsheets (1-10) including Motoring with a Wheelchair; Driving Licences; Insurance; Motoring Accessories.
RADAR Holiday Factsheets (1-13) including useful Addresses and Publications for the Disabled Holidaymaker; Holiday Insurance Cover; Planning and Booking A Holiday.

General
Care in the Air – available from The Secretary, Air Transport Users Committee, 2nd Floor,

Kingsway House, 103 Kingsway, London WC2B 6QX *tel* 071-242 3882.
Access to the Underground – A Guide for Elderly and Disabled People. Available 'over the counter' price 70p, at Travel Information offices or by post at £1 from: Unit for Disabled Passengers, London Regional Transport, 55 Broadway, London SW1H 0BD.
Stay on a Farm – A Guide to Farm and Country Holidays. Included is an index of establishments suitable for disabled people. Available through bookshops or Tourist Information Centres, price £5.95.
Tourism for All: a recent report from the English Tourist Board, looks at ways in which holiday opportunities for people with disabilities can be improved. The report makes recommendations to the tourist industry, Government and the Tourist Boards on improvements needed to accommodation, transport, attractions, and information provision to make holiday taking easier for people with special needs, with the aim of ensuring that they are catered for in the mainstream holiday market. Copies of the report are available from the English Tourist Board, 24 Grosvenor Gardens, London SW1W 0ET, price £5.00.
Door to Door. A guide to transport for disabled people. Published by the Department of Transport and available from Disabled Unit, Room F10/21 Department of Transport, Marsham Street, London SW1P 3EB.
Register of Swimming Clubs for Handicapped People. Available from: National Association of Swimming Clubs for the Handicapped, The Willows, Mayles Lane, Wickham, Hampshire PO17 5ND *tel* (0329) 833689.

Adaptation of Car Controls for Disabled People – Guidelines intended to help the many garages and individuals who are asked to convert vehicles to suit the needs of the disabled person. Copies of the guidelines are available from: Marion Blower, Institute of Mechanical Engineers, 1 Birdcage Walk, London SW1H 9JJ *tel* 071-222 7899 at a cost of £8.50 including postage and packaging.

USEFUL ADDRESSES

AA Information Centre, Leeds *tel* (0345) 500600.

British Association of Wheelchair Distributors, The Secretary, 1 Webbs Court, Buckhurst Avenue, Sevenoaks, Kent TN13 1LZ *tel* (0732) 458868.

Centre For Accessible Environment, 35 Great Smith Street, London SW1P 3BJ *tel* 071-222 7980. Information on accessibility and planning in public places and buildings.

Department of the Environment for Northern Ireland, Roads Service Headquarters, Commonwealth House, 35 Castle Street, Belfast BT1 1GU *tel* Belfast (0232) 321212.

Department of Transport, Marsham Street, London SW1P 3EB *tel* 071-276 3000.

Disability Scotland, Princes House, 5 Shandwick Place, Edinburgh EH2 4RG *tel* 031-229 8632; *fax* 031-229 5168. Produce two holiday directories (one covering Scotland, one the rest of the UK and abroad).

Disabled Drivers' Association, Ashwellthorpe Hall, Ashwellthorpe, Norwich, Norfolk NR16 1EX *tel* Fundenhall (050 841) 449.

Disabled Drivers' Motor Club, Cottingham Way, Thrapston, Northants NN14 4PL *tel* (0832) 734724; *fax* (0832) 733816.

Disabled Living Foundation, Information Service, 380-384 Harrow Road, London W9 2HU *tel* 071-289 6111.

Disabled Motorists Federation, National Mobility Centre, Unit 2a Atcham Estate, Upton Magna, Shrewsbury SY4 4UG *tel* (0743) 761889.

Holiday Care Service, 2 Old Bank Chambers, Station Road, Horley, Surrey RH6 9HW *tel* (0293) 774535.

Mobility Advice and Vehicle Information Service (MAVIS), Department of Transport, Transport & Road Research Laboratory, Crowthorne, Berkshire RG11 6AU *tel* Crowthorne (0344) 770456, or for information service only *tel* 071-276 5255. Provides information on all aspects of transport for people with disabilities, including personal assessment/evaluation on driving ability, advice on suitable car controls/adaptations. Range of vehicles available for test driving on private road system, each equipped with hand controls showing different driving systems and adaptations.

Motability, Gate House, West Gate, Harlow, Essex CM20 1HR *tel* (0279) 635666.

Disability Action (Northern Ireland), 2 Annadale Avenue, Belfast BT7 3UR *tel* (0232) 491011.

The Royal Association for Disability and Rehabilitation (RADAR), 25 Mortimer Street, London W1N 8AB *tel* 071-637 5400.

Sports Council, 16 Upper Woburn Place, London WC1H 0QP *tel* 071-388 1277.

Tripscope, 63 Esmond Road, London W4 1JE *tel* 081-994 9294. A nationwide telephone service providing free travel and transport information and advice for disabled and elderly people, and those who care for them.

Wales Council for the Disabled, Llys Ifor, Crescent Road, Caerphilly, Mid Glamorgan CF8 1XL *tel* (0222) 887325/6/7; *fax* (0222) 888702.

Whether you are a seasoned traveller clocking up thousands of miles a year, or simply setting out with your wheelchair for the first time, these pages will provide handy, at-a-glance hints and tips for travelling with confidence.

Advance planning is always the key to successful travelling, and Gerald Simonds Healthcare has compiled this section to help you travel with confidence at all times. As a company which is dedicated to providing the most progressive mobility equipment available, it is also committed to helping disabled people enjoy trouble-free travelling - at home or abroad.

Would you know how and where to contact your wheelchair dealer for spare parts in case of emergency in a foreign country? What if you get a puncture - do you know how to ask for help in Spanish? How do you make sure of an accessible parking space on the car deck of a cross-channel ferry? And what's the German for

Gerald Simonds Healthcare. A travel companion.

'wheelchair'? The simple checklist overleaf will help you avoid potential pitfalls, while the foreign glossary has been designed to provide a useful translation of key words and phrases relating to mobility and access.

Gerald Simonds Healthcare can also help you achieve and maintain greater independence by supplying the finest wheelchairs, advanced seating systems, power units and walking aids. All the products have been specially selected to work together to create complete mobility systems which offer the maximum level of comfort, reliability and ease of use.

The company's team of experts, including specialists in mobility and seating, can guide you through the range to help select the most appropriate solutions to your own particular needs. This exceptionally detailed advice before you buy, coupled with total after-sales support, ensures that you are always completely happy with your decision - not just at the time you buy, but for years to come.

SAMSON POWER DRIVE

"It's as though kerbs and awkward slopes didn't exist."

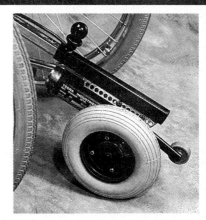

Does pushing your wheelchair exhaust you? Then Samson is the helper you need when you're out and about - to give you a push whenever the going gets tough.

Up a slope. Over a kerb. On the lawn. Or in the rough. He's there when you need him.

Samson is a small, light but powerful electric motor that fixes to the back of almost any folding wheelchair - just like an outboard on a boat. So simple. Easy to fix, easy to remove, Samson is your constant companion - wherever you go.

Samson comes in two versions: one for the active user to operate, and one for an attendant. You choose which is right for you.

For more details or a demonstration please call Gerald Simonds Healthcare on Aylesbury (0296) 436557. Do it now!

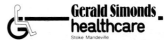

Gerald Simonds healthcare .
Stoke Mandeville

Gerald Simonds Healthcare Limited
9 March Place Gatehouse Way Aylesbury
Bucks HP19 3UG. Tel: 0296 436557

Sole British Isles distributor with a network of authorised dealers

Have wheels, will travel.

Travelling with your wheelchair can be problem-free as long as you prepare for the trip in advance. Don't be put off exploring by worrying about whether your wheelchair can go too - a few questions at the hotel, restaurant or tourist attraction will usually quickly and easily resolve any worries that you may have about facilities for disabled guests.

Long distance travel and foreign holidays do mean that you have to be particularly well organised both before you leave and during your stay. If you intend to do a lot of travelling abroad, always try your travel agent first for advice and information and be precise about your requirements and the facilities that you will need.

When travelling with your wheelchair, remember that not everyone is as familiar with it as you. You need to be confident that your wheelchair is in safe hands throughout the journey, but the baggage handler at a busy resort airport may not notice that one of the wheels is missing; the taxi driver may not know the best way to lift a wheelchair into the boot of his car.

You can help to minimise any problems which could crop up by referring to our simple checklist for trouble-free travelling. This covers three main areas - the preparations you should make before you leave and your contact with airlines and ferry operators - but remember that they are general guidelines which will help you make the most of your trip wherever, and however, you travel.

BEFORE YOU LEAVE...

- Check with the travel agent, airline or ferry company about facilities for disabled travellers at the hotel, the airport, ferry terminal and on board. Check that the accommodation is accessible and that you have details of the size of lifts, the position of the toilet in the hotel bathroom for easy transfer, the height of the bed, and access to the balcony or kitchen (if self-catering).

- Most airlines impose special conditions relating to electric wheelchairs but will carry them providing certain requirements are met. If you use an electric wheelchair, check with the airline well in advance and ask for consent in writing in case of any dispute at the check-in desk.

- Make sure that the couriers organising transfers between the airport and hotel are aware of your disability so that alternative transport can be arranged if necessary.

- Check that each part of your wheelchair is individually labelled if you are to be separated from it at any stage of the journey.

- Check the insurance on your wheelchair. Make sure it is adequately covered - most airline policies give insufficient cover of only £200 - £250.

- Consider having special puncture-proof tyres fitted before you leave. These will give you ease of mind and eliminate the need to spend time repairing a puncture, which can be a common and time-consuming problem in countries where the roads and pavements are not up to UK standards.

- Make sure that you have a puncture repair kit, tyre levers and a pump with you if you do not have puncture-proof tyres fitted.
A straightforward cycle kit is ideal and easy to use while spare inner tubes are always a good back-up. A small tool kit will enable you to make minor adjustments to your wheelchair quickly and easily.

- If you are travelling by car and have enough space, take a spare wheel for your chair in case of damage.

- Take your wheelchair-narrower with you, if you have one.

- Check before you leave that your dealer is able to supply any spare parts that you may need in an emergency. Take his address, telephone number and fax number with you.

- If you are at risk of pressure sores, remember to take additional protection for when you are out of your wheelchair. The small, lightweight Jay Protector cushion fits into a sling which can be strapped around your waist and legs to hold it firmly in place while you move about, and is ideal as a car and bath cushion.

WHEN YOU'RE FLYING...

- When checking in, be aware that despite prior notification, there may be a delay in organising a porter to help you transfer to the plane. Allow extra time for this.

- At most airports, you can stay in your own wheelchair until embarkation but some may ask you to transfer. If this is likely to cause discomfort, you can ask to stay in your own chair until boarding.

- Be aware that your chair may be thrown around a bit by baggage handlers. Ask for it to be put on board last. Ask the stewardess for it to be ready on the tarmac on arrival.

- If you need a special seat on the plane, perhaps close to the toilet or where there is more leg room, request this at the check-in desk otherwise seats will be allocated on a first come, first served basis.

- Don't leave your cushion on the chair - sit on it in the aircraft.

ON THE FERRY...

- If travelling by ferry, let them know in advance that you are coming, that you use a wheelchair and what assistance, if any, you will need. Put this in writing and keep a copy of the letter.

- Check that there is an adequate lift and a wheelchair-accessible toilet on board.

- When booking your crossing, check which operators offer concessions for disabled drivers.

- Most ferry companies ask disabled drivers to arrive an hour or more ahead of sailing time, so they may be placed at the front of the vehicle queue. Ask to be allowed to drive on first so you can park near the lift and get yourself and your chair out of the car in plenty of space.

- Many of the larger companies also give disabled travellers a sticker to put on their windscreen - this helps the loading officer to identify your car easily.

- Once on board, take your time to collect your belongings - there is no access to the car deck after sailing.

- If you have a long crossing to make, check that the ferry has some wheelchair-accessible cabins, close to a lift. Alternatively, book a reclining seat but check that you can reach this area in a wheelchair.

AND FINALLY ...

- Always check that hotel lifts, as well as doorways, are wide enough for your chair.

- On the flight, don't forget to remind the stewardess to radio ahead and arrange for assistance if necessary.

- Don't be reticent about demonstrating to airport staff and taxi drivers how your wheelchair works and/or folds.

Have a good trip!

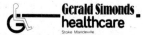

WORD PERFECT

At the airport/ on the plane	French	German	Spanish
May I have a wheelchair to take me to the aircraft please?	Pourrais-je avoir un fauteuil roulant pour me transporter jusqu' à l'avion s'il vous plaît?	Könnte ich einen Rollstuhl haben, um zum Flugzeug zu kommen?	Me peuden llevar al avión en silla de ruedas, por favor?
Please arrange for a wheelchair to meet the aircraft at...	Pourriez-vous faire en sorte qu'on vienne me chercher à l'avion avec un fauteuil roulant?	Bitte lassen Sie mich per Rollstuhl vom Flugzeug in/um ... abholen	Prepárenme una silla ruedas a la salida del avión en ...
Where is the nearest fire exit/toilet?	Où se trouve la sortie de secours/le wc la/le plus proche?	Wo ist der Nächste Notausgang/WC?	Dónde está la salida de incendios más cercana?/Dónde están los lavabos?
May I please have a seat with extra legroom?	Pourrais-je avoir un siège avec une place supplementaire pour les jambes?	Kann ich bitte einen fußfreien Sitz haben?	Puede darme un asiento con espacio adicional para las piernas, por favor?

At the ferry terminal/on board

Can I take the wheelchair on the boat?	Puis-je emporter le fauteuil roulant sur le bateau?	Kann ich den Rollstuhl auf das Schiff mit nehmen?	Puedo llevar la silla de ruedas en el barco?

Motoring

Please put the wheelchair in the car	Veuillez mettre le fauteuil roulant dans la voiture	Bitte tragen Sie meinen Rollstuhl in das Auto	Haga el favor de poner la silla de ruedas en el coche
This car is specially adapted for a disabled driver	Cette voiture est specialement adaptée pour un conducteur infirme	Dieses Auto ist für körperbehinderte Fahrer eingerichtet	Este coche está especialmente preparado para un conductor inválido
This car is hand controlled	Cette voiture est commandée manuellement	Dieses Auto wird handgesteuert	Este coche tiene los mandos en las manos
I have a disabled passenger	J'ai un passager infirme	Ich habe einen körperbehinderten Mitfahrer	Tengo un pasajero inválido
May I park here?	Puis-je parquer ici?	Darf ich hier parken?	Puedo estacionar aqui?
My car has broken down. Where is the nearest garage?	Ma voiture est en panne. Où est le garage le plus proche?	Mein Auto hat eine Panne. Wo Ist Die nächste Werkstätt?	Mi coche está cstropeado, Cuál es el garaje más próximo?

At the Hotel

Have you a room suitable for a person in a wheelchair?	Avez-vous une chambre appropriée à un infirme dans un fauteuil roulant?	Haben Sie ein Geeignetes Zimmer Für Einen Körperbehinderten mit Rollstuhl?	Tiene usted una habitación adecuada para una persona en silla de ruedas?
Are there any steps/stairs?	Y-a-t'il des marches/ des escaliers?	Sind hier Stufen/ Stiegen?	Hay escalones/ escaleras?
Is there a ramp/slope?	Y-a-t'il une rampe de montée/un plan incliné?	Ist dort eine Auffahrt/ein Hügel?	Hay una rampa/un terraplén?
Is there an entrance without steps?	Y-a-t'il une entrée sans marches?	Gibt es einen Eingang ohne Stufen?	Hay alguna entrada sin escalones?
Is there a lift (elevator)?	Y-a-t'il un ascenseur?	Gibt es einen Aufzug?	Hay ascensor?

Parts of a Wheelchair

Fork	Fourche	Gabel	Horquilla
Leg rest	Pose-jambes	Beinstütze	Estribo para la pierna
Foot plate	Pose-pieds	Fußplatte	Estribo
Wheel	Roue	Rad	Rueda
Hand rim	Pose-bras	Handstütze	Borde
Tyre	Pneu	Reifen	Cubierta
Castor	Gallet	Rolle	Ruedecilla
Battery/Motor	Baterie/Moteur	Batterie/Motor	Batería/Motor
Controller	Controlleur	Steuerknüppel	Mandos
Frame	Cadre	Gestell	Cuadro
Axle	Axe	Achse	Eje
Cushion	Coussin	Polster	Cojín
My/this ... is broken	Mon/ce ...est en panne	Mein/dies ... hat versagt	Mi/este ... está roto
Can you repair it/this for me?	Pourriez-vous me le réparer/me réparer ce?	Könnten sie mir es/das reparieren?	Puede usted reparármelo?
It is very urgent/important	C'est très urgent/important	Es ist sehr dringend/wichtig	Es muy urgente/importante
Where can I buy...?	Où puis-je acheter ...?	Wo kann ich ... kaufen?	Dónde puedo comprar ...?

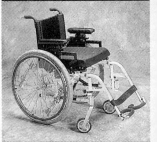
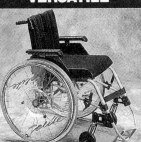
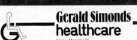

THE DISABLED TRAVELLER ABROAD

Choice is the key word when planning any holiday and there is no reason why, as a disabled person, you should not include overseas travel amongst the possibilities available. The Travel Trade, hoteliers, ferry operators and national tourist offices are showing increased awareness of the needs of the disabled person who wishes to travel abroad.

The onus is on disabled travellers to ensure that any special requirements are clearly understood by those who will be catering for them. To achieve this your most important contact is your travel agent who will be able to give advice and make sure that facilities you require are available. He can only do this if you co-operate by being completely frank about the nature of your disability and its effects including special diets and any routine which has to be followed to ensure good health.

Any misunderstanding, which can so easily arise without careful and detailed planning, can result in mistakes which may only come to light after you have started your holiday.

To assist in planning your trip abroad, here are some guidelines:

FORWARD PLANNING

1 Unless completely confident that you will not require assistance from anyone, either on the journey or at your holiday destination, it is advisable not to plan on travelling alone.
2 Consider the time of your proposed travelling, for excessive heat or cold can cause problems for disabled people.
3 Find out as much as possible about the area you wish to visit.

MAKING YOUR RESERVATIONS

It is advisable to let your Travel Agent deal with reservations after giving him detailed information about the limitations of your disability.

TRAVELLING BY SEA

Car carrying ferries and hovercraft offer a choice of routes out of Britain. To ensure a trouble free crossing, it is essential that the shipping company is made aware of any help you may need on the journey so that they can arrange for staff to be on hand to give necessary aid at terminals or on board the vessel. Shipping companies are becoming aware of the needs of the disabled person, and this awareness is being reflected in the design of new vessels and alterations carried out on those already in service.

ROUTE INFORMATION

The following facilities for the disabled have been inspected by the AA's hotel and restaurant inspectors and their reports and findings are contained in 'The AA Guide to Ferries', available free from AA shops.

Cairnryan-Larne
P&O European Ferries. Ships have lift, toilets, special parking and assistance available.

Dover-Boulogne
P&O European Ferries. Ships have a lift, toilets, special parking and assistance available.

Dover-Calais
P&O European Ferries. Ships have lifts, toilets, special parking and assistance available. Wheelchairs provided on The Pride of Dover. Advance notice required for special parking on The Pride of Bruges.

Sealink Stena Line. Lift and toilets on all shops. Access to all passenger areas on the Stena Fantasia and Stena Invicta and access to all seating areas on the Fiesta and Cote d'Azur.

Dover-Ostend
RMT (partner of P&O). The Reine Astrid has a lift and toilets. A new ship, the Prins Filip commenced service in the Autumn of 1991 and has not yet been inspected.

Felixtowe-Zeebrugge
P&O European Ferries. Ships have a lift, toilet and cabins.

Fishguard-Rosslare
Sealink Stena Line. The Stena Felicity has a lift, toilets, cabins and access to all seating areas.

Harwich-Hook of Holland
Sealink Stena Line. Ships have a lift, toilets, cabins and access to all seating areas.

Holyhead-Dun Laoghaire
Sealink Stena Line. The Stena Cambria has a lift, toilet and access to all seating areas.

Newhaven-Dieppe
Sealink Stena Line. Ships have lifts and toilets.

Ramsgate-Dunkerque
Sally Ferries. Ships have toilets and lifts giving access to all facilities on board.

Southampton to Cherbourg
Sealink Stena Line. The Stena Normandy has a lift, toilets and cabins.

Stranraer to Larne
Sealink Stena Line. Ships have lifts, toilets and access to all seating areas.

For further information the telephone numbers of the above ferry companies are shown below:

P&O European Ferries: (0304) 223000
Sealink Stena Line: (0233) 647022
RMT: (0304) 203388
Sally Ferries: (0843) 595522

Brittany Ferries
Brittany Ferries operate on the following routes:
Plymouth-Roscoff
Plymouth-Santander
Portsmouth-Caen
Portsmouth-St Malo
All ships are reported by our inspectors as having suitable lifts and cabins. For further information *tel* (0705) 827701.

NORTH SEA FERRIES
In the North Sea Ferries' terminal at Hull there are lifts between floors and special toilet facilities for the disabled. Ferries are accessible by wheelchair via the passenger walkways which have a graduated slope. For disabled passengers travelling by car, arrangements can be made (with prior notice) for the vehicle to park next to a lift on the car deck. If required, staff can be made available to take passengers on and off the ship.

Once on board there are lifts between all decks giving easier access for disabled passengers and upon request you can reserve one of the specially adapted cabins. These are situated on the same deck as the Purser's office and feature extra wide doors outside and inside to give easy access for wheelchairs and a special toilet/shower area with supports around the shower and toilet, a drop-down seat in the shower and low level wash basin. All of these cabins are fitted with an alarm button. There are three disabled cabins on each of the vessels on the Rotterdam service and one cabin on each of the vessels on the Zeebrugge service. The inside special cabin fare is charged for these cabins and they have to be booked in advance.

Enquiries and bookings: North Sea Ferries, King George Dock, Hedon Road, Hull HU9 5QA *tel* (0482) 77177.

CONCESSIONS FOR FERRIES

The majority of ferry companies offer varying concessions to the disabled driver on a wide variety of routes. However, it is emphasised that these concessionary schemes are very complex and varied, and are only available through full membership of the Disabled Drivers' Association, the Disabled Motorist's Federation or the Disabled Drivers' Motor Club, all of which will supply full information on the services and concessions available (see pages 130 for addresses). A disabled driver resident in the Republic of Ireland should contact the Disabled Drivers' Association of Ireland at the following addresses: Ballindine, Co. Mayo *tel* (094) 64266/64054; Carmichael House, 4 North Brunswick Street, Dublin 7 *tel* (01) 721671; South Terrace, Cork *tel* (021) 313033, or the Irish Wheelchair Association, Arus Chuchulain, Blackheath Drive, Clontarf, Dublin 3, *tel* 338241/2/3, for information on the services and concessions available between the Republic and Great Britain.

Sealink Stena Line offer reductions for all disabled passengers. For further information and booking refer to the Sealink Ferry Guide or write to: Sealink Stena Line, Reservations Department, Charter House, Park Street, Ashford, Kent TN24 8EX *tel* (0233) 647047.

THE CHANNEL TUNNEL

The Channel Tunnel is planned to open for traffic at the end of 1993. From that date "Le Shuttle" will provide a new means of crossing the Channel. By carrying cars inside purpose-built shuttle trains, the journey will become quicker and easier than ever before.

The service has been designed to cater for the needs of disabled passengers.

The terminals are linked directly to the motorways on each side of the Channel, the M20 in the UK and the new A16 in France. In these areas there will be a wide range of retail and catering outlets, including Duty-Free shopping.

Both British and French frontier controls will be carried out on the departure terminal before driving onto the shuttles. These will leave every 15 minutes at the busiest times, providing a no-booking service where you simply arrive and get on the next available departure. Arriving on the other side, drive straight onto the motorway and continue on your way.

Disabled travellers will have a special area of the shuttle in which to travel, where trained staff will be on hand to assist.

The overall journey time from leaving one motorway to joining the other will be just one hour, of which only 35 minutes will be spent crossing between the terminals.

TRAVELLING BY AIR

To make sure you are properly looked after, always tell the travel agent or airline when you make your booking that you have a special need, only eat certain foods, rely on the use of a wheel-chair or are disabled in some way.

Tell them if you need any help when you get to the airport or the terminal. Also ask if the airline makes any charge for special assistance such as an ambulance or wheelchair at airports en route to your destination. It is advisable to find out all the details about methods of transport to and from the aircraft and compare the arrangements of the various airlines before choosing an airline and making a booking.

You may be asked to get your doctor to fill in a form stating the nature of your disability and confirming you are able to travel.

Heathrow Airport (*tel* 081-759 4321)

There are special car parking bays provided at each of the short term car parks and passengers using wheelchairs are advised to use the bays which are located close to entrances and lifts. Long term car parks are provided with a special coach service for drivers with disabilities which is available on request. Parking on yellow lines by disabled drivers is not permitted anywhere on the airport.

London Transport operates frequent Airbus Services linking Heathrow's four terminals with various points in Central London. Buses operating on these services are adapted to carry two wheelchair passengers. For further details *tel* 071-227 3299.

Each terminal building is equipped with ramps and lifts which are usually located close to the stairs or escalators. Special toilet facilities for wheelchair travellers are clearly signed and public telephones in each terminal are accessible and at a suitable height.

Gatwick Airport (*tel* (0293) 535353)

For travellers arriving by rail, the local station manager can arrange for Gatwick Station staff to give assistance on arrival; further advice *tel* (0293) 524167. Disabled drivers are advised to seek advance information by calling one of the following numbers:

North Terminal – Europarks plc
(0293) 502737
South Terminal – APCOA Parking (UK) Ltd
(0293) 502896
Gatwick Airport Ltd – Car Parks Operations
(0293) 503899

Bays for orange badge holders are reserved in the multi-storey car parks of both terminals for short or long stay parking, giving level access into the terminal. A chauffeur-driven private car hire service is available with cars accessible to wheelchair-bound passengers, which can be booked in advance *tel* (0293) 562291.

For wheelchair passengers, ramps and/or lifts are provided where there is a change of level. Reserved seating is provided in the check-in area. Unisex toilets accessible to wheelchair-bound passengers are located throughout both terminals and telephones are push button and at suitable heights.

Birmingham Airport (tel (021) 767 5511)
For a stay less than four hours, spaces are reserved in the short stay car park close to the terminal building. For longer periods, spaces on the ground floor of the Multi-Storey car park are available, situated adjacent to the terminal building and accessible via a covered walkway. If assistance is required, press 'assist button' situated at the barrier control arm at the entrance/exit.

Toilets for disabled travellers are provided throughout the terminal building and also in the Multi-Storey car park. Keys held in control room of the car park.

Glasgow Airport (tel (041) 887 1111)
For disabled passengers arriving by bus, airport staff will give assistance from the bus to check-in desks. If driven by another person in a car, the driver will be able to stop briefly in front of the terminal, however, a policeman should be contacted first if the disabled passenger requires the driver to accompany them to the check-in. Disabled passengers taking their own cars will find spaces reserved for Orange Badge at the nearest point to the terminal. Arrangements can be made to get you to the terminal building by telephoning the Airport Duty Manager.

Access to the terminal is at pavement level through automatic doors. Disembarkation is at ground level as well as baggage reclaim and dispersal from the terminal. A new lift has been installed giving access to the duty free shop.

A wheelchair-accessible toilet is located on the ground floor, at the west end of the Check-in Hall and on the first floor on the main concourse and in the International Departures Lounge. Telephones in the terminal are available to wheelchair users at various locations. Refreshment areas are accessible by public lift.

Luton Airport (tel (0582) 405100)
Open air parking is available at the Airport. Disabled drivers are strongly recommended to write in advance to the Managing Director in order that special arrangements may be made to allow parking adjacent to the Terminal Building. Parking for disabled visitors in the Spectators Car Park (under 12 hours) is free, subject to an orange disabled badge being displayed.

All Terminal Building facilities are at ground floor level and have been designed with disabled travellers in mind. Ramps and automatic doors have been provided to ensure easy access to the Terminal Building.

Disabled toilet facilities are available in the Landslide Concourse, Departure Lounge and Arrivals Hall. Wheelchairs are available upon request at airline check-in desks. Specialised equipment is also available to help the disabled board the aircraft.

Stansted Airport (tel (0279) 680500)
Disabled passengers arriving by train can be met at Stansted Airport Railway Station. Arrangements can be made through the local station manager. The Coach Station is located in front of the Terminal Forecourt, giving easy access to and from the Terminal by lift and ramp. Reserved parking bays for orange badge holders are located in the Short Stay Car Park, close to the Terminal Entrance. Access into the Terminal is by lift or ramp. For assistance use the Courtesy Telephones provided next to the parking bays. There are frequent courtesy buses to and from the long stay car park to the Terminal. All are fitted with wheelchair lifts and tracking. If you use a wheelchair and require special parking assistance contact Ground Transportation at the airport.

Check-in islands in the Terminal are equipped with two low level desks, designed specifically for wheelchair users. Suitable toilets and push button telephones are located throughout the Terminal. In the Terminal all passenger facilities are on a single level and there are lifts from the rail and coach stations and Short Stay Car Park. Staff provide assistance on request in self-service shopping and catering areas.

YOUR HOLIDAY ACCOMMODATION

1   Show your Travel Agent the 'basic requirements' shown on page 41 in the Guide to assist him in finding suitable accommodation.
2   If you are seeking self-catering accommodation, an apartment or villa, ensure that it is suitably located and accessible.
3   There should be suitable level surroundings in the immediate environment of your accommodation.

MOTORING ABROAD

Any AA Shop will provide you with all the

information necessary for your European motoring holiday. As a first step you should consider the purchase of AA 5-Star Service. Available to both members and non-members, it is invaluable when travelling abroad. For further information and to discuss your particular requirements contact your local AA Shop.

MEDICAL TREATMENT ABROAD

Urgently needed medical treatment in the event of an accident or unforeseen illness can be obtained by most visitors, free of charge or at reduced cost, from the health-care schemes of those countries with whom the UK has health-care arrangements. Details are in the Department of Health (DH) booklet T4 which also gives advice about health precautions and vaccinations. Free copies are available from main post offices, the Health Publications Unit, No 2 Site, Manchester Road, Heywood, Lancs OL10 2PZ or by ringing 0800 555777. However, as the facilities and financial covers can differ considerably between the various countries, and the cost of bringing a person back to the UK is never covered under these arrangements, you are strongly advised to purchase a travel insurance policy such as AA Travelsure or 5-Star Personal.

Although the accommodation has not necessarily been inspected by the AA the following organisations are among those assisting in holidays abroad.

The Winged Fellowship arranges group holidays for disabled people to hotels and holiday centres abroad. It is necessary to book well in advance. Enquiries to: Winged Fellowship at their address on page 104.

Tenerife: 'Mar y Sol' Health and Fitness Resort, Los Cristianos. Purpose-built for wheelchair users. Totally accessible self-catering apartments and studios. Details available from the UK representative: Lynne James, 7 Overpool Road, Ellesmere Port, South Wirral L66 1JW *tel* 051-339 5316.

Camping for the Disabled is an organisation that acts as an information service for disabled campers. It is able to provide lists of accessible sites in France, Switzerland and West Germany, as well as Great Britain. Requests for suitable sites in Denmark, Netherlands, Norway, Spain and Sweden are also able to be dealt with, all for a small membership fee. Enquiries to: David G. Griffiths, Camping for the Disabled, 20 Burton Close, Dawley, Telford, Shropshire TF4 2BX *tel* (0743) 761889 & (0952) 507653.

REPUBLIC OF IRELAND

The following concessionary facilities are **only** available to disabled drivers **resident** in the Republic of Ireland. Principally these concessions take the form of an exemption from payment of road tax and a rebate of petrol duty.

Road Tax – Disabled drivers with specially adapted vehicles should apply to their local Motor Registration Office for the relevant application forms. The form should be returned duly completed together with the appropriate certificate completed by a member of the Garda Siochana confirming that the applicant's car has been converted for hand-control use. It should be noted that the concessionary facilities only apply to vehicles up to 2000 cubic centimetres. On the assumption that the items are found to be satisfactory by the local licensing authority, a tax exemption disc will be issued together with a statement from the authority to the effect that exemption has been granted in accordance with the appropriate legislation.

Petrol Rebate – Disabled drivers are entitled to Duty refund on petrol used. The present allowance is 600 gallons per year. In order to receive the rebate it is necessary to register as a disabled driver with Office of Revenue Commissioner, Petrol Rebate Section, 14-16 Lord Edward Street, Dublin 2.

Excise Duty – A disabled person importing a vehicle into the Republic is entitled to a full refund of the excise duty. All applications, giving details of the vehicle to be imported, should be directed to the Office of Revenue Commissioners, 14-16 Lord Edward Street, Dublin 2, accompanied by a doctor's certificate stating the exact disability.

Value-added Tax – A disabled person purchasing a new car which has been specially constructed or adapted for his use may obtain a repayment of the full amount of the value-added tax. The tax is paid at the time of purchase, but the Office of Revenue Commissioners, VAT Repayment

Section, 14-16 Lord Edward Street, Dublin 2, will advise as to how this may be recovered.

Grants — A grant may be obtained from your local Health Board towards the purchase of a car (but this is subject to a means test). This also applies to the disabled person who is unable to drive and requires a car to take him or her to and from work. Sympathetic consideration is also given to an applicant who requires a car for social purposes only. Applications can be made to the Chief Medical Officer or your local Health Board.

Parking concessions — A disabled person who drives a vehicle which is exempted from road tax may obtain exemption from payment of parking meter fees. Parking concessions are also available where there is a need to park in restricted areas in towns and cities. Application for these facilities should be made to the local authority.

Disabled drivers may display an adapted version of the International Symbol of Accessibility on their windscreens. This badge is only available from the Irish Wheelchair Association and is recognised as a parking badge by agreement with the police.

In Dublin, disabled drivers should also display the Dublin Corporation Parking Badge, this can be obtained by applying to the Corporation of Dublin, Traffic Department, 17-18 Christchurch Place, Dublin 8.

ORANGE BADGE SCHEME

Reciprocal arrangements with European countries

Holders of orange badges who visit countries which provide parking concessions for their own disabled citizens are able to take advantage of the concessions made by host countries by displaying their orange badge. Apart from the United Kingdom, some 12 countries are taking part in the scheme.

It should be noted that in some countries responsibility for introducing the concessions rests with individual local authorities. They may, therefore, not be generally available. In such cases badge holders should enquire locally, as they should whenever they are in any doubt as to their entitlement.

AUSTRIA

The Austrian scheme of parking concessions allows badge holders to park without time limit where sign C18 is used and they may stop (even where double parked) where sign C19 is displayed. Sign C19 is also used to indicate that badge holders may park in a pedestrian zone when loading and unloading is permitted.

Parking is also allowed without time limit at parking areas normally reserved for short-term parking.

Special parking places for disabled persons' vehicles may also be set aside near such places as hospitals and public service facilities for the care of people with disabilities.

BELGIUM

Badge holders may park without time limit where others may park only for a limited time and in parking places specifically reserved for disabled persons' vehicles. (These are indicated by sign E23 with an additional sign showing the disabled person symbol.)

Badge holders are exempt from paying at parking meters where local regulations explicitly provide for such payment.

DENMARK

Parking for up to 15 minutes is allowed:
— where only loading and unloading is permitted.
— where parking is prohibited, and
— on those parts of pedestrian areas where delivery vehicles are allowed.

Parking for up to one hour is allowed where 15 or 30 minutes parking is permitted.

Unlimited parking is allowed:
— where one, two or three hours parking is permitted (the time of arrival must be shown on a parking disc).
— at parking meters or car parks with coin machines, so long as the maximum amount is paid on arrival and the parking disc is set at the arrival time.

FINLAND

In order to obtain the parking concessions, a disabled visitor has to acquire a Finnish parking permit from the local police by presenting to them a parking permit granted in their own country. This permit must be displayed in a visible place inside the windscreen when the vehicle is parked.

Any badge holder granted a permit by the police is entitled to park, free of charge, in a parking space where parking is subject to payment and in an area where parking is prohibited by road signs, (C18 and C21) provided that other traffic regulations do not hinder it.

FRANCE

Responsibility for parking concessions in urban areas rests with the local (rather than regional or national) authorities.

Apart from reserved parking spaces for people with disabilities (indicated by the international symbol) there are no general street parking concessions. However, the police are required to show tolerant consideration for parking by identifiable disabled persons' vehicles – providing they are not causing an obstruction.

There are a number of local concessions which vary from town to town. In Paris, for example, disabled people are exempt from street parking charges, and benefit from a 75% reduction in car parking charges.

GERMANY

Badge holders are allowed to park:

- for a maximum of 3 hours where sign C18 is displayed (the time of arrival must be shown on a parking disc).
- beyond the permitted time in an area covered by sign C21.
- beyond the permitted time where sign E23 is displayed, or at pavement parking areas for which the parking period is restricted by a supplementary sign.
- during the permitted periods for loading and unloading in pedestrian zones.
- without charge or time limit at parking meters.

unless other parking facilities are available within a reasonable distance.

Reserved parking spaces for people with disabilities are also provided.

IRELAND

The badge issued to disabled drivers in the UK is recognised by the Irish authorities and should be displayed in a prominent position when visiting the Republic. However, the concessions only apply at parking meters and areas where parking discs are in operation; they do not entitle the driver to park on single or double yellow lines or areas where they are likely to cause an obstruction.

ITALY

Responsibility for the concessions rests with the local authorities. In general, public transport is given priority in town centres and private cars may be banned but the authorities are required to take special measures to allow badge holders to take their vehicles into social, cultural and recreational activity areas as well as their work places.

Reserved parking bays are provided, indicated by signs with the international symbol. (A small number of spaces are reserved for particular vehicles and in such cases the sign will show the appropriate registration number.)

LUXEMBOURG

In most urban areas reserved parking places are provided and indicated by signs C18 or E23 with the international symbol. Generally, badge holders are not allowed to exceed the parking time limit.

NETHERLANDS

Badge holders are entitled to the following concessions:

- the use of a car park set aside for handicapped people. (The parking place must be signed and there is no time limit.)
- indefinite parking in blue zones.
- indefinite parking at places marked with the E23 sign in conjunction with an additional panel stating parking time.
- parking at places marked with signs C18 and C20 for a maximum of 2 hours. A disabled person's parking disc must be used. The concession does not apply where other parking facilities exist within a reasonable distance.

PORTUGAL

Parking places are reserved for badge holders' vehicles. These are indicated by signs with the international symbol.

Badge holders are not allowed to park in places where parking is prohibited by a general regulation or a specific sign.

SWEDEN

Badge holders are allowed to park:

- for three hours where parking is banned or allowed only for a shorter period due to local regulations.
- for a period of 24 hours where a time limit of three hours or more is in force.

— in reserved parking spaces indicated by signs with the international symbol.

In general, parking charges must be paid although there might be local exemptions. The local police can give further information.

SWITZERLAND

Badge holders are allowed to park:
- for four hours where parking is restricted to 20 minutes or more, or within blue zones.
- for two hours where parking is prohibited altogether, or within red zones.
- these concessions only apply if there is no public or private parking place with unlimited parking time available to the public in the immediate vicinity of the parking place. Badge holders are also required to observe any special police restrictions, regulations in private parking places, traffic rights of way, parking time limits shorter than 20 minutes and no stopping zones.

Concessions at parking meters vary from town to town. Badge holders should enquire at a local police station to see whether concessions are available.

OTHER COUNTRIES

There are no formal reciprocal arrangements with **Norway**, but it is understood badge holders are allowed to park in ordinary meter or paying parking spaces free of charge and without time limit. They may also use spaces marked with signs 'reserved parking for disabled persons entitled to parking concessions' but these spaces may be subject to limitation.

In **Spain** most large towns and cities operate their own individual schemes but types of badges used and the concessions provided are not standardised. It is understood, however, that consideration would be shown to badge holders from other countries.

No schemes exist in **Gibraltar**, **Greece** or the former **Yugoslavia**.

OVERSEAS ORGANISATIONS

For those intending to travel abroad, the many national tourist offices in London are able to provide information on travel in their respective countries. In addition the following organisations will advise the handicapped tourist visiting their country, but any information received may not necessarily be in English.

AUSTRIA

Wiener Verkehrsverband, Obere Augartenstrasse 40, 1020 Vienna (0222) 211140.

Club Handikap, Interessensgemeinschaft der Behinderten, Taborstrasse 58/1, 1020 Vienna (0222) 4671045.

BELGIUM

Service du 'Car de l'Evasion', Comité Provincial de Namur, Croix-Rouge de Belgique, Rue de l'Industrie 124, B-5002 Saint-Servais (Namur) *tel* (081) 73 02 24.

DENMARK

DHF, Dansk Handicap Forbund, Kollektivhuset, Hans Knudsens Plads 1, 10, DK-2100, København *tel* 31293555.

PTU, Landsforeningen af Pollo-, Traflk- & Ulykkesskadede, Tuborgvej 5, 2900 Hellerup *tel* 31629000.

FINLAND

"Rullaten r.y," Vartiokyläntie 9, SF-00950 Helsinki *tel* 90-322069 or 326870 *fax* 90-326887.

FRANCE

Comité National Français de Liaison pour la Réadaptation des Handicapés, 38 Boulevard Raspail, 75007 Paris *tel* 4548 90 13.

GERMANY

Bundesarbeitsgemeinschaft Der Clubs Behinderter Und Jhrer Freunde, 6500 Mainz, Eupenerstrasse 5 *tel* (06131) 2255 or 225778.

Bundesuerband Selbsthilfe Körperbehinderter 7109 Krautheim/Jagst, Altkrautheimerstrasse 17 *tel* (06294) 68109 *fax* (06294) 68122.

ITALY

Centro Studi e Consulenza Invalidi, Via Gozzadini 7, 20148 Milan *tel* (02) 40308339 *fax* (02) 26861144.

NETHERLANDS

The Royal Dutch Touring Club ANWB Wassenaarseweg 220, PO Box 93200 2509 BA The Hague *tel* 070-314 7147. (A brochure 'Holland, The Handicapped' is available to readers by writing to The Netherlands Board of Tourism, 25-28 Buckingham Gate, London SW1E 6LD *tel* 071-931 0707 between 2pm and 4pm.

NORWAY

Norges Handikapforbund, PO Box 9217 Grøn-land, N-0134 Oslo 1 *tel* 02-170255. (Visitors address: Galleri Oslo Schweigaardsgt 12, 0134 Oslo 1).

PORTUGAL

Ministério do Emprego e Segurança Social, Secretariado Nacional de Reabilitação, Avenida Conde Valbom, 63-1000 Lisboa *tel* 7936517/ 7973537 *fax* 7965182.

SPAIN

Centro Estatal de Autonamía Personal y de Ayudas Técnicas, Los Extremeños, No 1, E-28038 Madrid *tel* 34-1-778.90.61 *fax* 34-1-778.41.17.

SWITZERLAND

Mobility International Schweiz, Hard 4, 8408 Winterthur *tel* (052) 256825 *fax* (052) 256838.

Swiss Invalid Association, Froburgstrasse 4, 4601 Olten *tel* 062 321 262 *fax* 062 323 105.

PUBLICATIONS USEFUL TO THE OVERSEAS TRAVELLER

The Disabled Traveller's Phrasebook Book 1, Western European Languages. This publication has been compiled specially to release the physically handicapped from the worry of language problems.

It contains a vocabulary of some 200 specialised phrases and over 50 phrases of particular importance to the disabled. The book is intended as a supplement to ordinary pocket dictionaries and phrasebooks which may be used in conjunction with it. The contents are listed under several main headings and a range of symbols have been designed to assist clarity and speed of reference.

Book 1 contains the following languages:

Dutch	Italian
English	Portuguese
French	Spanish
German	Swedish

Copies of the book and further information can be obtained from Disabled Drivers' Association, Ashwellthorpe Hall, Ashwellthorpe, Norwich, Norfolk NR16 1EX *tel* Fundenhall (050841) 449.

The following is a selection of the many publications available through RADAR. For an up-to-date price list write to the Royal Association for Disability and Rehabilitation, 25 Mortimer Street, London W1N 8AB, enclosing a large stamped addressed envelope.

Access in Paris
Access in Israel

Holidays and Travel Abroad: A Guide for Disabled People

For disabled drivers planning to visit the USA, the AAA have produced "The Disabled Drivers' Mobility Guide," which contains descriptive listings of driver/training facilities, adaptive equipment manufacturers, and organisations that provide other services to drivers with a handicap: This publication may be obtained from:

The American Automobile Association
Traffic Safety and Engineering Department
1000 AAA Drive
Heathrow, Florida 32746-5063
USA.

Prepayment is required; $5.95 plus shipping at time of going to press.

ACCOMMODATION

The following list of hotels can provide accommodation with at least one room suitable for the disabled.

Hotel Groups
It is possible to reserve accommodation at hotels belonging to hotel groups by contacting the hotel group on their reservation numbers:
Holiday Inns 071-722 7755
Hotel Ibis/Mercure/Novotel/Sofitel 071-724 1000.

Country/Town	Hotel	Rooms	Address/Telephone No.
AUSTRIA			
Innsbruck	Goldener Adler		Herzog-Friedrichstr 6 *tel* (0512) 586334
	Ibis		Schützenstrasse 43 *tel* (0512) 65544
	Maria Theresia		Maria-Theresienstrasse 31 *tel* (0521) 5933
Salzburg	Europa		Rainerstr 31 *tel* (0662) 889930
Wien (Vienna)	Ibis		Mariahilfer Gürtel 22-24 *tel* (0222) 565626
BELGIUM			
Antwerpen (Anvers)	Switel		Copernicuslaan 2 *tel* (03) 2316780
Brugge (Bruges)	Novotel	2	Chartreuseweg 20 *tel* (050) 38 28 51
Brussel (Bruxelles)	Ibis		Grasmarkt 100, Rue de Marche Aux Herbes *tel* (02) 5144040
	Novotel	2	Rue du Marche Aux Herbes 120 *tel* (02) 5143333
Gent (Gand)	Holiday Inn		Ottergemsesteenweg 600 *tel* (091) 225885
	Novotel	3	Gouden Leeuwplein 5 *tel* (091) 242230
Liége (Luik)	Hotel Urbis	2	Centre Opéra, 41 Place de la Republique Française *tel* (041) 236085
DENMARK			
Aalborg	Limfjordshotellet		Ved Stranden 14-16 *tel* 98164333
Kobenhavn (Copenhagen)	Imperial		Vester Farimagsgade 9 *tel* 33128000
	SAS Royal		Hammerischsgade 1 *tel* 33141412

Country/Town	Hotel	Rooms	Address/Telephone No.
Kolding	Tre Roser		Dyrehavegårdsvej Byparken *tel* 75532122
Odense	HC Andersen		Claus-Bergsgade 7 *tel* 66147800

FRANCE

Country/Town	Hotel	Rooms	Address/Telephone No.
Aix-en-Provence	Ibis	2	Chemin des Infirmeries *tel* 42279820
Aix-en-Provence −Beaumanoir	Novotel	2	Résidence Beaumanoir Autoroute A8 *tel* 42274750
Aix-en-Provence −Sud	Novotel	2	Avenue Arc de Meyran *tel* 42279049
Bourg-en-Bresse	Ibis	3	Boulevard Charles de Gaulle *tel* 74225266
Caen	Novotel	4	Avenue Côte de Nacre *tel* 31930588
Caen (Hérouville St Clair)	Ibis	3	4 Quartier Savary *tel* 31956000
	Campanile	2	Parc Tertiarie Boulevard du Bois *tel* 31952924
Calais	Campanile	2	rue de Maubeuge Zac du Beau Marais *tel* 21343070
Chalon-sur-Saòne	Campanile	2	Rue Raoul Ponchon *tel* 85412324
	Mercure	2	Avenue de l'Europe *tel* 85465189
Dijon	Campanile	2	1 rue de la Fleuriée Saint Apollinaire *tel* 80724538
Dijon - Sud	Ibis	2	R.N. 74 Route de Lyon, Perrigny-les-Dijon *tel* 80528645
	Novotel	2	Route de Beaune (RN74) *tel* 80521422
Evry	Ibis	4	1 Avenue du Lac Parc Tertiaire du Bois-Briard Courcouronnes *tel* 60777475
Fontainebleau	Ibis	3	18 rue de Ferrare *tel* 64234525
Genéve Aéroport (France)	Novotel	2	Route de Meyrin *tel* 50408523
Genéve - Ferney Voltaire	Campanile	2	Chemin de la Planche Brûlée *tel* 50407479
Lançon/Provence	Mercure	1	Autoroute A7 *tel* 90428711

Country/Town	Hotel	Rooms	Address/Telephone No.
Le Havre	Mercure	4	Chaussée d'Angouléme *tel* 35212345
Le Harve-Gonfreville	Campanile	2	Zone d'activités du Camp Dolent *tel* 35514300
Lille	Royal	20	2 Boulevard Carnot *tel* 20510511
Lille-Lomme	Novotel	3	Autoroute A25 - Sortie Lomme 7 *tel* 20070999
Lille - Sud	Campanile	2	rue Jean-Charles-Borda *tel* 20533055
Lyon Bron	Novotel	6	Avenue Jean-Monnet 260 *tel* 78269748
	Campanile	2	rue Maryse Bastié *tel* 78264540
	Ibis	4	36 Avenue du Doyen Lepine *tel* 78543134
Lyon-Ecully	Campanile	4	42 Avenue Guy de Collongue *tel* 78331693
Lyon - Est Beynost	Ibis	1	Les Baterses Autoroute A42 sortie N5 *tel* 78554088
Lyon - Gerland	Ibis	6	Les Berges du Rhone 68 Avenue Leclerc *tel* 78583070
Lyon - Nord	Ibis	3	Autoroute A6 - Porte de Lyon *tel* 78660220
Lyon - Part-Dieu	Mercure	4	47 Boulevard Vivier-Merle *tel* 72341812
Lyon - Part-Dieu Sud	Ibis	4	Place Renaudel *tel* 78954211
Lyon - Sainte Foy	Campanile	2	35 Chemin de la Croix Pivort *tel* 78593223
Mâcon - Nord	Novotel	4	Autoroute A6 - Péage Mâcon Nord, Sennece-les-Mâcon *tel* 85360080
Mâcon - Sud	Campanile	2	ZAC des Bouchardes *tel* 85374141
	Ibis	2	Les Bouchardes - Chaintre *tel* 85365160
Nice - Cap 3000	Novotel	2	40 Avenue de Verdun *tel* 93316115
Nice - Promenade des Anglais Aeroport	Ibis	3	Promenade des Anglais 359 *tel* 93833030
Nîmes	Campanile	2	Chemin de la Careiras *tel* 66842705
	Ibis	4	Parc Hotelier, Ville Active *tel* 66380065
	Novotel	4	Esplanade Charles-de-Gaulle *tel* 66765656

Country/Town	Hotel	Rooms	Address/Telephone No.
Nîmes - Ouest	Mercure	1	Rue Tony Garnier, Ville Active *tel* 66841455
PARIS Aulnay-Sous-Bois	Novotel	2	R.N. 370 *tel* 48662297
Le Bourget	Novotel	2	2 rue Jean-Perrin Le Blanc-Mesnil *tel* 48674888
Cergy-Pontoise	Novotel	2	3 Avenue du Parc *tel* 30303947
La Défense	Novotel	12	2 Boulevard de Neuilly Defense 1 *tel* 47781668
Ermont-Sannois	Campanile	2	rue des Loges *tel* 34137957
Massy-Palaiseau	Novotel	2	18/20 rue Emile Baudot Zone d'Activité *tel* 69208491
Meulan	Mercure	3	Lieu-dit 'Ile Belle' *tel* 34746363
Montesson	Campanile	2	9 rue du Chant des Oiseaux *tel* 30716334
Montmarte	Mercure	7	3 rue Caulaincourt *tel* 42941717
Montrouge/Porte D'Orléans	Mercure	5	13 rue François Ory *tel* 46571126
Porte de Pantin	Mercure	4	25 rue Scandici, Pantin *tel* 48467066
Porte de Plaine	Mercure	9	rue du Moulin. Vanves *tel* 46429322
Saclay	Novotel	2	Rue Charles-Thomassin *tel* 69356600
St Germain-en-Laye	Campanile	2	Route de Mantes - R.N. 13 Maison Forestiére *tel* 34515959
Les Ulis/Orsay	Mercure	2	3 rue Rio Solado Z.A. de Courtaboeuf *tel* 69076396
Reims	Campanile	2	Echangeur A4 Saint-Rémy, Accés Avenue Georges Pompidou Val de Murigny II *tel* 26366694
Reims-Est	Mercure	2	Route de Châlons *tel* 26050008
Reims-Tinqueux	Novotel	3	Route de Soisson (N31) *tel* 26081161
Rouen	Ibis	2	56 Quai Gaston Boulet *tel* 35704818
Rouen – Sud	Ibis	3	2 Avenue Maryse-Bastié *tel* 35660363

Country/Town	Hotel	Rooms	Address/Telephone No.
Rouen – Sud	Novotel	2	Le Madrillet *tel* 35665850
Strasbourg-Centre Halles	Novotel	4	Quai Kléber *tel* 88221099
Strasbourg Sud	Campanile	2	20 rue de l'ill, Geispolsheim *tel* 88667477
	Mercure	2	rue du 23 Novembre - Ostwald Illkirch-Graffenstaden *tel* 88673200
	Novotel	2	R.N. 83 Route de Colmar *tel* 88662156
Tours – Joué-les-Tours	Campanile	2	Route de Chinon Avenue du Lac Les Bretonnières *tel* 47672489
Tours – Nord	Hotel Ibis	3	La Petite Arche Avenue Maginot *tel* 47543220
Tours – Sud	Campanile	2	Rue de la Berchottière *tel* 47279500
	Hotel Ibis	3	R.N. 10 'La Vrillonnerie' *tel* 47282528
	Novotel	4	R.N. 10 – Zac de la Vrillonnerie *tel* 47274138
Valenciennes	Campanile	2	Valenciennes Aérodrome *tel* 27211012
	Novotel	2	Zone Industrielle No 2 Autoroute Paris-Bruxelles *tel* 27442080

GERMANY

Country/Town	Hotel	Rooms	Address/Telephone No.
Aachen	Ibis		Friedlandstrasse 6-8 *tel* (0241) 47880
	Novotel	1	Am Europaplatz *tel* (0241) 16870
Bonn - Hardtberg	Novotel	2	Konrad Adenauer-Damm/Max Habermannstr 2 *tel* (0228) 25990
Dortmund – West	Holiday Inn		Olpe 2 *tel* (0231) 543200
	Novotel	2	Brennaborstrasse 2 *tel* (0231) 65485
Hamburg – Nord	Novotel	2	Oldesloerstrasse, 166 *tel* (040) 5502073
Köln – West	Novotel	2	Horbellerstrasse 1 *tel* (02234) 5140
Mannheim	Holiday Inn		Kurfürstenarkade N6 *tel* (0621) 10710

Country/Town	Hotel	Rooms	Address/Telephone No.
Mannheim	Novotel	2	Auf dem Friedensplatz 1 *tel* (0621) 42340
	Intercity Mannheim		Im Hauptbahnhof *tel* (0621) 1595-0
Marl	Novotel	2	Eduard-Weitsch-Weg 2 *tel* (02365) 1020
Munich (München)	Arcade		Dachauerstrasse 21 *tel* (089) 551930
	Mercure	2	Senefeldersh 9 *tel* (089) 551320
Oberstdorf Rubi	Viktoria	6	Riedweg 5 *tel* (08322) 4583
Saarbrücken	Novotel	2	Zinzingerstrasse 9 *tel* (0681) 58630
	Pullman Kongress		Hafenstr 8 *tel* (0681) 30691
	Residence		Faktoreistr 2 *tel* (0681) 38820

ITALY

Country/Town	Hotel	Rooms	Address/Telephone No.
Aosta	Valle d'Aosta		Corso Ivrea 146 *tel* (0165) 41845
Bergamo	Excelsior San Marco		Plaza della Repubblica 6 *tel* (035) 232132
Milan (Milano) Ca' Granda	Ibis		Viale Suzzani 13 *tel* (02) 66103000
	Novotel	4	Viale Suzzani *tel* (02) 66101861
Prato	President		Via Simintendi 20 *tel* (0574) 30251
Roma	Holiday Inn		via Aurelia Antica 415 *tel* (06) 6642
Siena	Villa Scacciapensieri		via Scacciapensieri 10 *tel* (0577) 41441

NETHERLANDS

Country/Town	Hotel	Rooms	Address/Telephone No.
Amsterdam	Grand Krasnapolsky		Dam 9 *tel* (020) 5549111
Amsterdam Airport	Barbizon Schiphol		Kruisweg 495 Schiphol *tel* (020) 6550550
Amersfoort	Berghotel		Utrechtseweg 225 *tel* (033) 620444
Dordrecht	Postiljon		Rijksstraatweg 30 *tel* (078) 184444
Heereuveen	Postiljon		Schaus 65 *tel* (05130) 24041
Hoogeveen	Baron Hoogeveen		Mathysenstrasse 1 *tel* (05280) 63303
Maarsbergen	Maarsbergen		Woudenbergseweg 44 *tel* (03433) 1341

Country/Town	Hotel	Rooms	Address/Telephone No.
Nijmegen	Altea Nijmegen		Stationsplein 29 *tel* (080) 238888
Putten	Postiljon		Strandboulevard 3 *tel* (03418) 56464
Rotterdam	Hilton		Weena 10 *tel* (010) 4144044
SPAIN			
Barcelona	Majestic		Paseo de Gracic 70 *tel* (93) 4881717
Madrid	Holiday Inn		Plaza Carlos Trias, Breton 4 *tel* (01) 5970102
	Novotel	4	Albacete 1 *tel* (01) 4054600
Seville (Sevilla)	Meliá Sevilla		Avienda Eduardo, Dato 49 *tel* (95) 4570040
	Porta Coeli		C/Dr Pedro Castro 1 *tel* (95) 4422611
SWITZERLAND			
Basel (Bâle)	Basel Hilton		Aeschengraben 31 *tel* (061) 2716622
Bern	Savoy		Neuengasse 26 *tel* (031) 224405
	Schweizerhof		Bahnhofpl 11 *tel* (031) 224501
Genève (Geneva)	Holiday Inn		26 Voie de Moëns *tel* (022) 7910011
	President		47 quai Wilson *tel* (022) 7311000
Interlaken	Lac		Höheweg 225 *tel* (036) 222922
Lausanne	Royal Savoy		av d'Ouchy 40 Ouchy *tel* (021) 264201
	Paix		av de Benj-Constant 5 *tel* (021) 207171
Lugano	International au Lac		via Nassa 68 *tel* (091) 227541
Luzern (Lucerne)	Carlton-Tivoli		Haldenstrasse 57 *tel* (041) 513051

FRENCH 'AUTOROUTE' (MOTORWAY) SERVICE AREAS

The following 'autoroute' (motorway) service areas with facilities for the disabled are listed as a general guide and derived from the publication 'LA FRANCE DES AUTO-ROUTES pour les usagers à mobilité réduite'. Facilities shown include Hotel (H), Buffet Bar (B), Restaurant (R) and Toilet (T). Service Stations are available at all service areas shown unless otherwise stated i.e. No S/Sta. Many Buffet Bars and Restaurants shown will have toilets for disabled people included, but we cannot verify these facilities from the information provided. In addition, access to a service area shop and/or telephone is possible at most service areas.

LOCATION	FACILITIES FOR THE DISABLED	LOCATION	FACILITIES FOR THE DISABLED
A1 Paris – Lille 215 km	**NORTHBOUND**	**A1 Lille – Paris 215 km**	**SOUTHBOUND**
Vemars *(26 km Paris)*	B, R, T	Phalempin *(200 km Paris)*	R, T
Ressons *(81 km Paris)*	R	Asservillers *(122 km Paris)*	H, R
Asservillers *(122 km Paris)*	H, B, R	Ressons *(81 km Paris)*	R
Croisilles *(157 km Paris)*	T	Vemars *(26 km Paris)*	H, R, T
Phalempin *(200 km Paris)*	R, T		
A2 Bapaume – Crespin 62 km	**NORTHBOUND**	**A2 Crespine – Bapaume 62 km**	**SOUTHBOUND**
No facilities for disabled people		La Sentinelle *(56 km Bapaume)*	B
A4 Paris – Strasbourg 487 km	**EASTBOUND**	**A4 Strasbourg – Paris 487 km**	**WESTBOUND**
Ussy Sur Marne *(57 km Paris)*	B	Lienbach *(442 km Paris)*	T, No S/Sta
Vrigny *(130 km Paris)*	B	Saverne-Monswiller *(432 km Paris)*	B
Reims Champagne *(160 km Paris)*	*B*	Katzenkopf *(414 km Paris)*	T, No S/Sta

LOCATION	FACILITIES FOR THE DISABLED	LOCATION	FACILITIES FOR THE DISABLED

A4 Paris – Strasbourg 487 km	EASTBOUND	A4 Strasbourg – Paris 487 km	WESTBOUND
Le Mont de Charme *(186 km Paris)*	T, No S/Sta	Longeville Les Saints-Avold *(352 km Paris)*	B, R
Valmy Orbeval *(206 km Paris)*	B	Brouck *(344 km Paris)*	T, No S/Sta
Rarecourt *(233 km Paris)*	T, No S/Sta	Metz St Privat *(305 km Paris)*	B
Charly Oradour *(320 km Paris)*	T, No S/Sta	Jubécourt *(233 km Paris)*	T, No S/Sta
		La Noblette *(186 km Paris)*	T, No S/Sta
Longeville Les Saints-Avold *(352 km Paris)*	B, R	Reims Champagne *(160 km Paris)*	R
Schalbach *(414 km Paris)*	T, No S/Sta	Gueux *(130 km Paris)*	B
		Le Tardenois Nord *(97 km Paris)*	R
		Bussy-Saint-Georges *(27 km Paris)*	B

A6 Paris – Lyon 460 km	SOUTHBOUND	A6 Lyon – Paris 460 km	NORTHBOUND
Les Lisses *(22 km Paris)*	R	Taponas *(408 km Paris)*	R
Villiers *(65 km Paris)*	T, No S/Sta	Les Sablons *(397 km Paris)*	T, No S/Sta
Nemours *(74 km Paris)*	R	Mâcon La Salle *(375 km Paris)*	H, R
Bois Des Chataigniers *(115 km Paris)*	T, No S/Sta	Saint Ambreuil *(342 km Paris)*	H
La Réserve *(123 km Paris)*	R	La Loyere *(323 km Paris)*	T, No S/Sta
Venoy Grosse Pierre *(167 km Paris)*	H, R	Beaune-Merceuil *(311 km Paris)*	H, R
La Couée *(185 km Paris)*	T, No S/Sta	La Repotte *(269 km Paris)*	T, No S/Sta
La Chaponne *(213 km Paris)*	R	Les Lochères *(256 km Paris)*	R
Chien Blanc *(256 km Paris)*	R	Maison Dieu *(213 km Paris)*	R
Chaignot *(269 km Paris)*	T, No S/Sta	Hervaux *(199 km Paris)*	T, No S/Sta
Beaune-Tailly *(311 km Paris)*	H, R	Venoy Soleil Levant *(167 km Paris)*	H, R
Curney *(323 km Paris)*	T, No S/Sta	Les Patures *(145 km Paris)*	T, No S/Sta

LOCATION	FACILITIES FOR THE DISABLED	LOCATION	FACILITIES FOR THE DISABLED

A6 Paris – Lyon 460 km	**SOUTHBOUND**	**A6 Lyon – Paris 460 km**	**NORTHBOUND**
La Ferté *(342 km Paris)*	R	La Couline *(123 km Paris)*	R
Mâcon Saint Albin *(375 km Paris)*	R	Floée *(86 km Paris)*	T, No S/Sta
		Darvault *(74 km Paris)*	R
Creches *(397 km Paris)*	T, No S/Sta	Villabé *(22 km Paris)*	R
Dracé *(408 km Paris)*	R		

A7 Lyon – Marseille 315 km	**SOUTHBOUND**	**A7 Marseille – Lyon 315 km**	**NORTHBOUND**
Solaize *(15 km Lyon)*	B, R	Vitrolles *(291 km Lyon)*	B
St Rambert Est *(60 km Lyon)*	B, R, T	Lançon *(273 km Lyon)*	B, R
		Noves *(231 km Lyon)*	T, No S/Sta
Portes-Les-Valence *(109 km Lyon)*	B, R, T	Sorgues *(215 km Lyon)*	B, R
Montelimar Ouest *(151 km Lyon)*	B, R, T	Mornas-Les-Adrets *(187 km Lyon)*	B, R
Mornas-Village *(189 km Lyon)*	R, T	Tricastin *(173 km Lyon)*	T, No S/Sta
Morières *(226 km Lyon)*	R	Montelimar Est *(151 km Lyon)*	H, B, R, T
Senas *(250 km Lyon)*	T, No S/Sta	Portes-Les-Valence *(109 km Lyon)*	B, R, T
Lançon *(273 km Lyon)*	H, B, R	St Rambert Ouest *(60 km Lyon)*	H, B, R, T
		Solaize *(15 km Lyon)*	B, R

A8 Aix-en-Provence – Menton 221 km	**SOUTHBOUND**	**A8 Menton – Aix-en-Provence 221 km**	**NORTHBOUND**
L'Arc *(38 km Aix-en-Provence)*	B	La Scoperta *(210 km Aix-en-Provence)*	B
Cambarette *(67 km Aix-en-Provence)*	R	Les Breguieres Nord *(168 km Aix-en-Provence)*	B, R
Roudai *(85 km Aix-en-Provence)*	T, No S/Sta	Le Canaver *(128 km Aix-en-Provence)*	R
Vidauban Sud *(106 km Aix-en-Provence)*	B, R	Candumy *(85 km Aix-en-Provence)*	T, No S/Sta

LOCATION	FACILITIES FOR THE DISABLED	LOCATION	FACILITIES FOR THE DISABLED
A8 Aix-en-Provence – Menton 221 km	**SOUTHBOUND**	**A8 Menton – Aix-en-Provence 221 km**	**NORTHBOUND**
Esterel *(143 km Aix-en-Provence)*	B	Cambarette Nord *(67 km Aix-en-Provence)*	R
Piccolaret *(166 km Aix-en-Provence)*	T, No S/Sta	Rousset *(38 km Aix-en-Provence)*	B
Les Breguieres Sud *(168 km Aix-en-Provence)*	R	Ventabren Nord *(8 km Aix-en-Provence)*	T, No S/Sta
A8–A52–A50 Chateauneuf le Rouge – Toulon 69 km	**SOUTHBOUND**	**A8–A52–A50 Toulon – Chateauneuf le Rouge 69 km**	**NORTHBOUND**
Le Pas d'Ouiller *(30 km Chateauneuf Le Rouge)*	T, No S/Sta	No facilities for disabled people	
A9 Orange – Le Pethus (Spain) 277 km	**SOUTHBOUND**	**A9 Le Perthus (Spain) – Orange 277 km**	**NORTHBOUND**
Travel Nord *(18 km Orange)*	B, R, T	Le Village Catalan *(165 km Orange)*	H, B, R
Vergeze Nord *(59 km Orange)*	T, No S/Sta	Lapalme *(218 km Orange)*	R, T
Montpellier – Fabrègues *(111 km Orange)*	H, R	Béziers – Montblanc *(154 km Orange)*	B, T
Narbonne – Vinassan *(182 km Orange)*	H, R	Vergeze Sud *(67 km Orange)*	T
Le Village Catalan *(265 km Orange)*	H, B, R	Roquemaure Sud *(10 km Orange)*	T
A10 Paris – Bordeaux 560 km	**SOUTHBOUND**	**A10 Bordeaux – Paris 560 km**	**NORTHBOUND**
Le Heron Cendré *(75 km Paris)*	T, No S/Sta	Saugon Est *(506 km Paris)*	B, R, T
Orleans Saran *(90 km Paris)*	R	Saint-Leger Est *(456 km Paris)*	B, R
Blois Villerbon *(143 km Paris)*	R	Les Ruralies *(372 km Paris)*	H, B, R
Maille *(251 km Paris)*	T, No S/Sta	Nouâtre *(251 km Paris)*	T, No S/Sta

LOCATION	FACILITIES FOR THE DISABLED	LOCATION	FACILITIES FOR THE DISABLED
A10 Paris – Bordeaux 560 km	**SOUTHBOUND**	**A10 Bordeaux – Paris 560 km**	**NORTHBOUND**
Chatellerault Antran (265 km Paris)	R	Tours Val de Loire (196 km Paris)	R
Les Ruralies (372 km Paris)	H, B, R	Blois Meners (143 km Paris)	R
Saint-Leger Ouest (456 km Paris)	B, R	La Dauneuse (75 km Paris)	T
Saugon Ouest (506 km Paris)	B, R	Limours Briis Sous Forges 5 km Paris)	B, R
A11 Ablis – Nantes 355 km	**WESTBOUND**	**A11 Nantes – Ablis 355 km**	**EASTBOUND**
Chartres – Gasville (52 km Ablis)	R	Varades La Bedoire (316 km Ablis)	B
Brou Frazé (99 km Ablis)	B	Baune Est (248 km Ablis)	T, No S/Sta
La Ferté Bernard (136 km Ablis)	R	Parcé sur Sarthe (211 km Ablis)	T
Pruillé Le Chetif (181 km Ablis)	T, No S/Sta	Sarges-les-Le Mans (166 km Ablis)	R
Parcé sur Sarthe (211 km Ablis)	T	Villaines La Gonais (136 km Ablis)	R
Varades Les Genetais (316 km Ablis)	B	Brou Dampierre (99 km Ablis)	B
		Chartres – Bois – Paris (52 km Ablis)	R
A81 Le Mans – Rennes 153 km	**WESTBOUND**	**A81 Rennes – Le Mans 153 km**	**EASTBOUND**
Saint-Denis D'Orques (248 km Paris)	B	Laval Le Goudray (276 km Paris)	B
Laval Bonchamp (276 km Paris)	B		
A13 Paris – Caen 227 km	**WESTBOUND**	**A13 Caen – Paris 227 km**	**EASTBOUND**
Morainvilliers (27 km Paris)	R	Beuzeville (171 km Paris)	B
		Bosgouet (128 km Paris)	R

LOCATION	FACILITIES FOR THE DISABLED	LOCATION	FACILITIES FOR THE DISABLED
A13 Paris – Caen 227 km	**WESTBOUND**	**A13 Caen – Paris 227 km**	**EASTBOUND**
Rosny-sur-Seine *(51 km Paris)*	R	La Villeneuve en Chevrie *(59 km Paris)*	T, No S/Sta
Vironvay *(93 km Paris)*	R	Morainvilliers *(27 km Paris)*	R
Robert Le Diable *(119 km Paris)*	T, No S/Sta		
Giberville *(220 km Paris)*	B		
A25 Lille – Dunkerque 77 km	**WESTBOUND**	**A25 Dunkerque – Lille 77 km**	**EASTBOUND**
St Laurent *(29 km Lille)*	B	St Eloy *(29 km Lille)*	B
A26 Arras – Calais 112 km	**NORTHBOUND**	**A26 Calais – Arras 112 km**	**SOUTHBOUND**
Villefleur *(46 km Calais)*	T, No S/Sta	Grand Riez *(46 km Calais)*	T, No S/Sta
A31 Thionville – Beaune 331 km	**SOUTHBOUND**	**A31 Beaune – Thionville 331 km**	**NORTHBOUND**
L'Obrion *(272 km Beaune)*	R	Gevrey – Chambertin *(25 km Beaune)*	B
Toul Dommartin *(228 km Beaune)*	H, R	Combe Suzon *(88 km Beaune)*	T, No S/Sta
Faverosse *(211 km Beaune)*	T, No S/Sta	Langres – Noidant *(103 km Beaune)*	R
Lorraine/La Trelle *(182 km Beaune)*	R	Bois de Chaumont *(162 km Beaune)*	T, No S/Sta
Montigny Le Roi *(138 km Beaune)*	B	Lorraine Les Rappes *(182 km Beaune)*	R
Côte Robert *(122 km Beaune)*	T, No S/Sta	Malvaux *(211 km Beaune)*	T, No S/Sta
Langres – Perrogney *(103 km Beaune)*	B, R	Loisy *(272 km Beaune)*	B
Dijon – Brognon *(56 km Beaune)*	R		
La Tille *(44 km Beaune)*	T, No S/Sta		
Gevrey – Chambertin *(25 km Beaune)*	R		

LOCATION	FACILITIES FOR THE DISABLED	LOCATION	FACILITIES FOR THE DISABLED

A36 Mulhouse – Beaune 230 km	WESTBOUND
Le Vieux Charmont *(47 km Mulhouse)*	T, No S/Sta
La Combe Ronde *(60 km Mulhouse)*	B
Pelousey *(129 km Mulhouse)*	T, No S/Sta
Saint Jean-de-Losne *(185 km Mulhouse)*	T, No S/Sta
Glanon *(201 km Mulhouse)*	R

A36 Beaune – Mulhouse 230 km	EASTBOUND
Sampans *(172 km Mulhouse)*	T, No S/Sta
Marchaux *(112 km Mulhouse)*	H, R
Chevaney *(102 km Mulhouse)*	T, No S/Sta
Ecot *(60 km Mulhouse)*	B
La Forêt *(27 km Mulhouse)*	T, No S/Sta
La Porte D'Alsace *(11 km Mulhouse)*	R

A40 Mâcon – Passy 200 km	EASTBOUND
Ceignes – Cerdon *(130 km Passy)*	R
Sylans *(116 km Passy)*	T, No S/Sta
Nangy *(50 km Passy)*	T, No S/Sta
Bonneville *(35 km Passy)*	R

A40 Passy – Mâcon 200 km	WESTBOUND
Bonneville *(35 km Passy)*	R
Valleiry *(79 km Passy)*	R, T
St Andre de Bage *(197 km Passy)*	T, No S/Sta

A41 Grenoble – Genève 150 km	NORTHBOUND
Mouxy *(98 km Grenoble)*	R
Les Crets Blancs *(144 km Grenoble)*	B

A41 Genève – Grenoble 150 km	SOUTHBOUND
Fontanelles *(126 km Grenoble)*	R

A43 Lyon – Albertville 143 km	EASTBOUND
Saint Priest *(8 km Lyon)*	B, R
L'Isle d'Abeau Sud *(28 km Lyon)*	H, R
Granier *(100 km Lyon)*	R
Val Gelon *(120 km Lyon)*	B

A43 Albertville – Lyon 143 km	WESTBOUND
Manissieu *(8 km Lyon)*	

LOCATION	FACILITIES FOR THE DISABLED	LOCATION	FACILITIES FOR THE DISABLED
A61 Toulouse – Narbonne 150 km EASTBOUND		**A61 Narbonne – Toulouse 150 km** WESTBOUND	
Port Lauragais *(41 km Toulouse)*	H, R	Les Corbieres *(108 km Toulouse)*	B
Belvedere de La Cité *(92 km Toulouse)*	T, No S/Sta	Belvedere d'Auriac *(92 km Toulouse)*	T, No S/Sta
Les Corbieres *(108 km Toulouse)*	B	Port Lauragais *(41 km Toulouse)*	H, R
A62 Bordeaux – Toulouse 252 km EASTBOUND		**A62 Toulouse – Bordeaux 252 km** WESTBOUND	
Le Bazadais Sud *(51 km Bordeaux)*	B	Frontonnais Nord *(207 km Bordeaux)*	R
Agen Porte d'Aquitaine Sud *(115 km Bordeaux)*	R	Agen Porte d'Aquitaine Nord *(115 km Bordeaux)*	R
Moirax *(128 km Bordeaux)*	T		
Garonne Sud *(161 km Bordeaux)*	B		
Frontonnais Sud *(207 km Bordeaux)*	R		
A63 Bordeaux – Hendaye 219 km SOUTHBOUND		**A63 Hendaye – Bordeaux 219 km** NORTHBOUND	
Labenne Ouest *(20 km St Geours-de-Marenne)*	B	Bidart Est *(48 km St Geours-de-Marenne)*	B
Bidart Ouest *(48 km St Geours-de-Marenne)*	B	Labenne Est *(48 km St Geours-de-Marenne)*	B

INDEX